THE SOUTH BEACH DIET OF 2025

The Ultimate Guide to Effortless Weight Loss Through Simple and Healthy Cooking

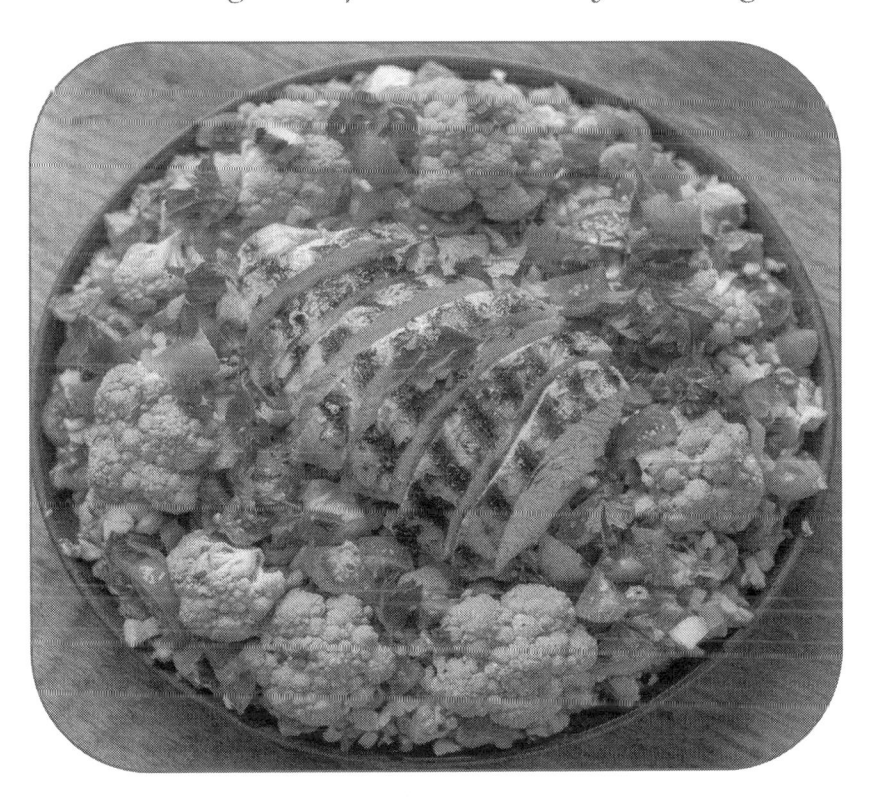

KRISTY NOLAN

Copyright©2025 Kristy Nolan

All Rights Reserved
No portion of this book may be reproduced in any form without permission from the publisher, except as permitted by U.S. copyright law.

TABLE OF CONTENTS

INTRODUCTION 5
   ABOUT THE AUTHOR: KRISTY NOLAN'S JOURNEY 5
      Understanding the South Beach Diet Revolution 6
      Why This Book is Different 7

PART ONE: THE SOUTH BEACH DIET FOUNDATION 8

CHAPTER 1 9
   THE SCIENCE BEHIND SOUTH BEACH DIET 9
      Understanding the Glycemic Index 9
      How Your Body Processes Food 10
      Why Traditional Diets Fail 11

CHAPTER 2 13
   THE THREE PHASES EXPLAINED 13
      Phase 1: Reset Your Body 13
      Phase 2: Steady Weight Loss 14
      Phase 3: Maintaining Your Success 16
      Transitioning Between Phases 17
      Final Thoughts on the Three Phases 18

CHAPTER 3 19
   SETTING UP YOUR SOUTH BEACH KITCHEN 19
      Essential Ingredients 19
      Kitchen Tools and Equipment 23
      Meal Planning Basics 24
      Smart Shopping Guide 25

CHAPTER 4 27
   LIFESTYLE STRATEGIES FOR SUCCESS 27
      Exercise Recommendations 27
      Creating a Routine 28
      Portion Control 30
      Building Healthy Habits 32

PART TWO: THE RECIPES 34

CHAPTER 5 35
   PHASE 1 RECIPES (TWO 35
   WEEK RESET) 35
      Breakfast Recipes 35
      Lunch Recipes 45

Korean-Style Beef Bowl with Cauliflower Rice 50
Approved Snacks 56
14-Day Meal Plan 56

CHAPTER 6 65

PHASE 2 RECIPES (STEADY LOSS) 65
Breakfast Recipes 65
Lunch Recipes 77
Dinner Recipes 87
Approved Snacks 98
14-Day Meal Plan 98

CHAPTER 7 107

PHASE 3 RECIPES (MAINTENANCE) 107
Lunch Recipes 118
Dinner Recipes 129
Approved Snacks 140
Meal Plans (14-Day Plan) 140

PART THREE: MASTERING THE LIFESTYLE 144

CHAPTER 8 145

COMMON MYTHS AND FACTS 145
Debunking Popular Diet Myths 145
Success Stories 148
Troubleshooting Guide 150

CHAPTER 9 153

FREQUENTLY ASKED QUESTIONS 153
General Diet Questions 153
Recipe Modifications 155
Special Dietary Needs 158
Weight Loss Plateaus 159

CONCLUSION 161

YOUR LIFELONG JOURNEY 161
Staying Motivated 161
Resources and Support 163
Final Thoughts 165
A Thank You Note from Kristy Nolan 167
🎁 CLAIM YOUR EXCLUSIVE BONUSES! 168

WEIGHT LOSS TRACKER & 30-DAYS WELLNESS TRACKER 170

The South Beach Diet Of 2025 | 4

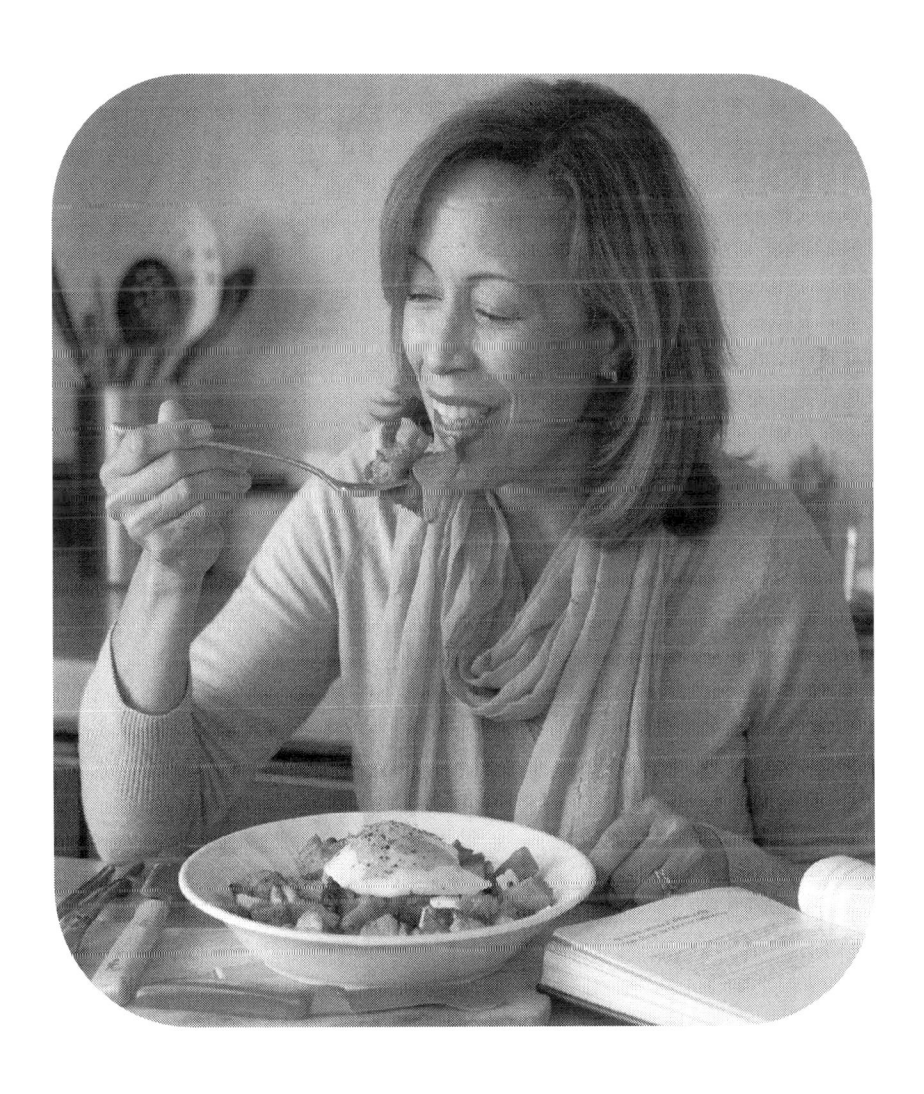

INTRODUCTION
About the Author: Kristy Nolan's Journey

Kristy Nolan never imagined she'd become the face of a transformative health movement. She was just like any other busy professional, juggling career demands and family responsibilities while trying to stay healthy. But her wake-up call came one sunny afternoon when she found herself out of breath after a short walk to her mailbox. It wasn't just the physical exhaustion—it was the realization that her energy, confidence, and zest for life had dwindled.

At that moment, Kristy decided she had to make a change—not just for herself but for her family. The quest for a sustainable solution led her to the South Beach Diet. The simplicity of its principles, combined with its emphasis on real, satisfying food, resonated deeply. For Kristy, it wasn't about a quick fix or fitting into a smaller dress size. It was about reclaiming her vitality and creating a lifestyle that didn't feel like a constant struggle.

Through trial and error, Kristy developed a unique approach to the South Beach Diet, adapting it to her life's demands without sacrificing flavor or enjoyment. Over the years, she not only achieved her health goals but also inspired friends and family to join her journey. This book is her way of sharing what she's learned—because Kristy believes everyone deserves to feel empowered, healthy, and confident in their own skin.

Understanding the South Beach Diet Revolution

The South Beach Diet isn't just another fleeting trend; it's a game changer for anyone tired of yo-yo dieting and endless calorie counting. At its core, the South Beach Diet is about resetting your relationship with food. It focuses on consuming the right carbohydrates and healthy fats while teaching your body to thrive on nutritious, satisfying meals.

The diet's revolutionary approach lies in its balance. Instead of cutting out entire food groups or forcing you into unrealistic restrictions, it helps you make smarter choices. Imagine eating a hearty breakfast, a delicious lunch, and a mouthwatering dinner—all while losing weight and feeling energized. That's the magic of South Beach.

Kristy remembers her early days on the diet vividly. The first two weeks, known as Phase 1, were a revelation. She remembers that although it wasn't easy, it wasn't horrible. "I was seeing genuine progress, and I wasn't starving." She learned the power of resetting her body's chemistry and overcoming bad desires during those first few days. As she transitioned through the phases, she realized this wasn't just a diet—it was a sustainable way of life.

The South Beach Diet also stood out because it encouraged flexibility. Kristy didn't have to give up the joy of eating out or celebrating special occasions. Instead, she learned how to navigate those situations with confidence. The more she lived it, the more she realized that this wasn't just a diet; it was a revolution in how we approach health and weight loss.

Why This Book is Different

Why yet another work about the South Beach Diet? you may ask. The answer is simple: this one is special. It's not just a collection of recipes or a rehash of the diet's principles. It's a heartfelt guide designed to make your journey as seamless and enjoyable as possible.

Kristy has walked the same path you're about to embark on. She knows the doubts, the slip-ups, and the small victories that make it all worth it. That's why this book is filled with practical tips, relatable stories, and real-life advice that goes beyond what most diet books offer.

The recipes in this book have been tested and perfected for busy lives. Whether you're a parent juggling kids' schedules, a professional with limited time, or someone just starting their health journey, these meals will fit into your life—not the other way around.

But it's not just about food. This book dives into the lifestyle changes that make the South Beach Diet work in the long run. From grocery shopping hacks to surviving social gatherings, Kristy shares everything she wishes someone had told her when she started.

Most importantly, this book is about you. It's about empowering you to take charge of your health without feeling overwhelmed or deprived. Kristy's hope is that by the time you turn the last page, you'll feel ready—not just to start the South Beach Diet but to embrace it as a lifelong friend.

Welcome to your fresh start. Let's make it count!

PART ONE: THE SOUTH BEACH DIET FOUNDATION

CHAPTER 1
The Science Behind South Beach Diet

Understanding the Glycemic Index

The glycemic index (GI) is a simple yet powerful concept that lies at the heart of the South Beach Diet. At its core, the GI measures how quickly a carbohydrate-containing food raises your blood sugar levels. Foods with a high GI, like white bread and sugary snacks, cause a rapid spike in blood sugar. This sudden rise triggers your body to release large amounts of insulin, which can lead to energy crashes, hunger pangs, and weight gain over time.

On the other hand, foods with a low GI, such as vegetables, beans, and whole grains, have a slower, steadier impact on blood sugar. They provide consistent energy and help keep hunger at bay. The South Beach Diet focuses on incorporating more low-GI foods into your meals, allowing your body to burn fat efficiently while maintaining stable energy levels.

Kristy Nolan, the author of this guide, remembers her "aha" moment when she first learned about the glycemic index. "I realized that the foods I was eating were working against me, even though I thought they were healthy," she adds. Once she started choosing lower-GI options, her energy improved, her cravings subsided, and the weight began to come off effortlessly.

How Your Body Processes Food

Understanding how your body processes food can make all the difference in your weight loss journey. Every meal you eat is broken down into three main components: carbohydrates, fats, and proteins. Each one plays a specific role in how your body generates energy, builds tissue, and stores fat.

Carbohydrates are your body's primary energy source. When you eat carbs, they're converted into glucose (sugar) and absorbed into your bloodstream. Your body stores extra glucose as fat if you ingest more than it needs.

Fats are essential for many bodily functions, including hormone production and cell repair. But it matters what kind of fat you eat. Healthy fats, like those in avocados and nuts, are beneficial, while trans fats and excessive saturated fats can harm your health.

Proteins are your body's building blocks. They aid in muscular growth, tissue healing, and prolonging feelings of fullness.

The South Beach Diet teaches you to balance these macronutrients in a way that supports weight loss and overall health. By choosing the right kinds of carbs, fats, and proteins, you can fuel your body effectively without feeling deprived.

Kristy shares her personal struggle with carb-heavy meals before discovering the diet. "Everything changed when I started incorporating lean proteins and healthy fats into my meals. I wasn't just losing weight—I felt amazing!"

Why Traditional Diets Fail

If you've tried dieting before, you're not alone. Most people have been through the cycle of restrictive eating, initial weight loss, and eventual regain. But why do traditional diets fail so often? The answer lies in their unsustainable approach.

- *Too Much Restriction*

Many diets rely on severe calorie cuts or the elimination of entire food groups. While this might lead to short-term results, it's hard to maintain in the long run. Deprivation leaves you feeling hungry, frustrated, and more likely to binge.

- *Lack of Flexibility*

Being on a diet does not mean that your life is over. Celebrations, holidays, and social events often derail strict eating plans. Traditional diets don't teach you how to navigate these situations, leading to feelings of failure when you **cheat.**

- *Ignoring Long-Term Habits*

Diets often focus solely on the number on the scale, ignoring the importance of building sustainable habits. Without learning how to shop, cook, and eat in a way that fits your lifestyle, it's easy to revert to old patterns once the diet ends.

The South Beach Diet stands apart because it addresses these pitfalls. Instead of focusing on what you can't have, it emphasizes delicious, nutrient-dense foods that you'll actually enjoy eating. Additionally, it promotes manageable, incremental adjustments as opposed to significant overhauls.

Kristy understands the frustration of failed diets. "Even though I would really begin with the best of intentions, after everything I would always end up starting afresh". The South Beach Diet felt different from the start—it wasn't about punishing myself but learning how to eat smarter."

With this diet, you're not just following rules—you're learning skills that will last a lifetime. And that's the real secret to success.

The South Beach Diet Foundation equips you with the science and tools you need to succeed. By understanding how your body processes food, making smarter choices, and avoiding the traps of traditional diets, you'll be on the path to lasting weight loss and vibrant health.

CHAPTER 2
The Three Phases Explained

The South Beach Diet is built on a three-phase structure designed to guide you from resetting your body to achieving sustainable weight loss and maintaining it for the long term. Each phase serves a specific purpose, working together to create a lifestyle that's realistic, effective, and enjoyable. Let's dive into the details of each phase and how to transition smoothly between them.

Phase 1: Reset Your Body

Phase 1 is the most structured part of the South Beach Diet. It's a two-week reset meant to kickstart your weight loss journey by stabilizing blood sugar levels, reducing cravings, and teaching your body to rely on fat for energy instead of sugar.

You'll cut out high-glycemic items like pasta, white bread, and sugary snacks during this phase. Instead, your meals will focus on lean proteins, healthy fats, and non-starchy vegetables. The goal isn't starvation—it's about nourishing your body with foods that promote fat burning and help you feel satisfied.

What You'll Eat: Think grilled chicken, turkey, fish, eggs, leafy greens, broccoli, cauliflower, avocados, and nuts. These foods are not only low on the glycemic index but also rich in nutrients.

What to Avoid: Say goodbye to refined carbs, fruit, alcohol, and sugary treats during this phase. These items can spike blood sugar and make it harder for your body to transition into fat-burning mode.

The book's author, Kristy Nolan, remembers her initial encounter with Phase 1. "I initially believed it would be impossible to give up bread and sweets," she admits. However, my cravings vanished and I felt more energized in a matter of days. It was about finding better options, not about deprivation.

Phase 1 also assists in resolving any form of emotional eating habits. By focusing on what your body truly needs, you start to see food as fuel rather than a quick fix for stress or boredom.

Key Benefits of Phase 1:
- You lose weight rapidly as your body shifts to burning fat.
- Reduced cravings for sugar and carbs.
- Improved energy levels and focus.

Phase 2: Steady Weight Loss

After two weeks in Phase 1, you'll move into Phase 2, where the focus shifts to steady, sustainable weight loss. This phase is less restrictive, allowing you to reintroduce some of the foods you avoided earlier—like fruits, whole grains, and dairy—in moderation.

What You'll Eat: Along with Phase 1 staples, you'll enjoy foods like berries, apples, quinoa, brown rice, and low-fat yogurt. These additions make meals more versatile and enjoyable while keeping blood sugar levels stable.

What to Avoid: While you can add more variety, you'll still need to avoid high-glycemic foods like white bread, sugary desserts, and processed snacks.

The beauty of Phase 2 is that it teaches balance. You'll learn how to incorporate carbs back into your diet without overdoing it. This phase is also about listening to your body — understanding what works for you and adjusting as needed.

According to Kristy, Phase 2 marked a sea change in her path. "I discovered my rhythm here," she says. "I no longer felt as though I was following a diet. All I was doing was eating what was healthy for my body and my life.

Key Benefits of Phase 2:
- Gradual, consistent weight loss that's easier to maintain.
- More diverse food options to keep meals engaging.
- Building long-term habits that support a healthy lifestyle.

Tips for Success in Phase 2:
Keep experimenting with recipes to find meals you love.
Stay mindful of portion sizes, especially with reintroduced foods.

Don't rush the process—Phase 2 is about steady progress, not quick fixes.

Phase 3: Maintaining Your Success

Phase 3 is the final stage of the South Beach Diet. By now, you've reached your goal weight or are close to it. The focus shifts from weight loss to maintaining your success and enjoying the healthy habits you've built.

This phase is the least restrictive, allowing you to eat all food groups in moderation. The principles you've learned in Phases 1 and 2—like choosing low-glycemic carbs, eating lean proteins, and incorporating healthy fats—remain the foundation of your diet.

What You'll Eat: Everything is on the table, but the emphasis remains on whole, nutrient-dense foods. You can occasionally enjoy a slice of cake or a glass of wine, but these should be treats rather than staples.

What to Avoid: There's no "off-limits" list, but you'll want to steer clear of falling back into old habits. Regular indulgence in sugary, processed, or high-GI foods can undo your progress.

Kristy considers how her connection with food evolved as a result of Phase 3. "I started enjoying my life and no longer worried about each bite," she says. "I was capable of taking pleasure in meals guilt-free due to the fact that I knew enough to make smart decisions."

Key Benefits of Phase 3:
- A sustainable way of eating that fits into any lifestyle.
- Freedom to enjoy occasional indulgences without losing control.
- Long-term health and weight maintenance.

Transitioning Between Phases

Transitioning between phases is an important part of the South Beach Diet journey. It's not just about changing what's on your plate—it's about shifting your mindset and adapting to new habits.

- *From Phase 1 to Phase 2:*

The transition from Phase 1 to Phase 2 is exciting because you get to reintroduce some of your favorite foods. Start slowly by adding one or two items at a time, like a small serving of fruit or a portion of whole grains. This helps you monitor how your body reacts and ensures you stay on track.

During this time, Kristy advises keeping a meal log. She suggests writing down what you eat and how you're feeling. "It enables you to identify certain trends and adjust as you deem necessary."

- *From Phase 2 to Phase 3:*

Moving into Phase 3 is a celebration of how far you've come. By this point, healthy eating should feel natural, not forced.

Continue practicing mindful eating and keep low-GI foods as the foundation of your meals.

Remember, transitioning doesn't mean abandoning the principles you've learned. Each phase builds on the last, creating a seamless path to lifelong health.

Final Thoughts on the Three Phases

The South Beach Diet's phased approach is what makes it so effective. Instead of overwhelming you with drastic changes, it guides you step by step, allowing your body and mind to adjust along the way.

Kristy's experience with the three stages is evidence of its effectiveness. According to her, "it wasn't just about me losing weight—it was more about gaining energy, confidence, and a clear, new perspective to life."

Whether you're just starting Phase 1 or settling into Phase 3, remember that every step you take brings you closer to your goals. Trust the process, and enjoy the journey. You're not just following a diet—you're building a healthier, happier you.

CHAPTER 3
Setting Up Your South Beach Kitchen

Starting the South Beach Diet means not only changing your eating habits but also transforming your kitchen into a space that supports your health goals. Setting up your kitchen is the first step to making this journey easier and more enjoyable. Whether you're a seasoned cook or just getting started, creating a well-stocked kitchen can make meal prep simpler and more efficient. Let's dive into how you can set up your South Beach kitchen to set yourself up for success.

Essential Ingredients

A well-stocked kitchen is key to following the South Beach Diet successfully. The right ingredients will help you prepare meals that are both delicious and aligned with the diet's principles. Here's a breakdown of the essential ingredients you'll need to have on hand.

Proteins

A key component of the South Beach Diet is protein. They help stabilize blood sugar, promote satiety, and are essential for muscle building.

Lean Meats: Chicken, turkey, and lean cuts of beef (like sirloin or tenderloin) are all great options. These are excellent sources of protein without excess fat.

Fish: Salmon, tuna, cod, and tilapia are not only rich in protein but also provide heart-healthy omega-3 fatty acids.

Eggs: Eggs are a cheap and adaptable source of protein. Opt for cage-free, organic eggs when possible.

Tofu and Tempeh: For plant-based protein, tofu and tempeh are great choices, providing all the essential amino acids your body needs.

Shellfish: Shrimp, crab, and other shellfish are low in fat and carbs, making them perfect for the South Beach Diet.

Vegetables

Vegetables should be the star of your meals, especially non-starchy ones. They help you consume less calories while providing fiber, vitamins, and minerals.

Leafy Greens: Spinach, kale, romaine lettuce, and arugula are great for salads, smoothies, or sautéing.

Cruciferous Vegetables: Brussels sprouts, cauliflower, and broccoli are rich in minerals and fiber.

Other Non-Starchy Veggies: Zucchini, bell peppers, cucumbers, asparagus, and mushrooms are low in calories and high in fiber.

Tomatoes: Tomatoes add flavor and nutrition to salads, soups, and sauces.

Healthy Fats

Fats are important on the South Beach Diet, but the focus is on healthy fats. These fats help with satiety, support metabolism, and are good for your heart.

Olive Oil: Extra virgin olive oil is a key source of healthy fats. Use it for cooking or as a base for dressings.

Avocados: Avocados are rich in monounsaturated fats and fiber, making them perfect for salads, spreads, or smoothies.

Nuts and Seeds: Almonds, walnuts, chia seeds, and flaxseeds are great snack options and can be added to salads, yogurt, or smoothies.

Nut Butters: Natural peanut butter or almond butter (without added sugars) are great for spreading on vegetables or whole grain crackers.

Whole Grains

While the South Beach Diet limits refined carbs, it still allows for certain whole grains. These grains provide fiber and essential nutrients.

Quinoa: A complete protein, quinoa is an excellent grain that is both gluten-free and rich in fiber.

Brown Rice: Brown rice is less processed than white rice and retains more of its natural nutrients.

Oats: Oats can be used for oatmeal or in baked goods.

Whole Wheat: When you reintroduce grains in Phase 2, whole wheat pasta or bread made from whole grains can be a healthy option.

Dairy and Dairy Alternatives

Dairy provides calcium and other essential nutrients, but it's important to choose low-fat or non-fat options.

Low-Fat Dairy: Choose non-fat or 1% milk, Greek yogurt, and reduced-fat cheese. These provide protein and calcium without excess fat.

Dairy Alternatives: If you're lactose intolerant or prefer plant-based options, consider almond milk, coconut milk, or soy milk.

Spices, Herbs, and Condiments

Flavors are important, and the South Beach Diet encourages the use of fresh herbs and spices. Avoid processed sauces and dressings that are high in sugar or unhealthy fats.

Herbs: Basil, cilantro, parsley, and thyme are great additions to any meal.

Spices: Cumin, turmeric, paprika, and garlic powder can enhance flavor without adding extra calories.

Condiments: Opt for mustard, hot sauce, and salsa. Avoid sugary ketchup and store-bought dressings.

Sweeteners

While sugar is off-limits, there are some alternative sweeteners you can use in moderation.

Stevia: A natural sweetener that doesn't spike blood sugar levels.

Erythritol: A sugar alcohol that's low in calories and doesn't raise blood sugar.

Xylitol: Another sugar alcohol, though it should be consumed in moderation.

Kitchen Tools and Equipment

With the right ingredients in hand, the next step is to equip your kitchen with the necessary tools to make meal prep easier. You don't need a fancy kitchen full of gadgets—just the basics that will help you prepare healthy, flavorful meals.

Essential Cooking Tools
Sharp Knives: A good set of knives is essential for chopping vegetables, slicing meat, and prepping food. A chef's knife, paring knife, and serrated knife will cover most needs.
Cutting Boards: Use separate cutting boards for meats and vegetables to avoid cross-contamination. Select ones that can be cleaned easily and are long-lasting.
Non-Stick Skillets: A quality non-stick skillet makes cooking proteins and vegetables easier while requiring less oil.
Saucepan: A medium-sized saucepan is perfect for cooking grains like quinoa or simmering sauces.
Baking Sheets: Baking sheets are great for roasting vegetables and cooking lean meats like chicken breasts.
Blender or Food Processor: A blender is essential for making smoothies, while a food processor can help you prepare soups, sauces, or chopped vegetables in no time.

Measuring Tools
Measuring Cups and Spoons: Accurate measurements help keep your portion sizes on track. These are especially important in the early phases of the diet when you're learning how much of each food to eat.
Kitchen Scale: A kitchen scale helps you measure portions of protein and other foods accurately.

Storage Containers
Having a variety of storage containers will help you organize your kitchen and store leftovers.

Glass Containers: Glass containers are ideal for storing prepped meals, leftovers, or snacks. They're reusable, easy to clean, and microwave-safe.
Plastic Bags and Wraps: These are useful for freezing individual portions of food like chicken breasts, fish fillets, or chopped vegetables.
Mason Jars: Perfect for making salads in a jar, smoothies, or storing dry ingredients like nuts and seeds.

Meal Planning Basics

Meal planning is an essential part of the South Beach Diet. With the right planning, you can make the diet fit into your busy schedule and avoid the temptation of unhealthy foods. Here are some basic steps to follow when planning your meals.

1. Plan Your Meals Around Protein and Veggies

Focus on lean proteins and vegetables when planning your meals. A typical South Beach meal should have a serving of protein, a non-starchy vegetable, and a healthy fat source. For example, grilled chicken with steamed broccoli and a drizzle of olive oil is a simple and balanced meal.

2. Prep Ahead of Time

Every week, set aside some time to prepare the ingredients. Grain cooking, protein marinating, and vegetable washing and chopping. This will help you maintain your diet and save you time throughout the week.

3. Batch Cook

One of the best ways to ensure that you have nutritious meals on hand is to cook in large quantities. Make a pot of quinoa, roast a large number of vegetables, or bake multiple chicken breasts at once. For convenient access, you can keep these in the refrigerator or freezer.

Mix and Match

Don't feel like you need to stick to a rigid meal plan. You can mix and match ingredients based on what's in your fridge or pantry. For example, leftover roasted chicken can be added to a salad, wrapped in a lettuce leaf, or served with quinoa for a quick meal.

Smart Shopping Guide

Knowing what to buy at the grocery store is crucial to setting yourself up for success. Here's how to shop smart while sticking to the principles of the South Beach Diet.

1. Stick to the Perimeter

The perimeter of the store is where you'll find the freshest foods—produce, lean proteins, dairy, and healthy fats. Focus on filling your cart with these items, and try to avoid the inner aisles where processed foods tend to lurk.

2. Shop Seasonal

Seasonal, fresh produce is typically more affordable and has a greater flavor. Plan your meals around what's in season to keep things interesting.

3. Buy in Bulk

Buy protein sources, grains, and nuts in bulk to save money and reduce packaging waste. Just remember to store them correctly to keep them fresh.

4. Read Labels

When you do buy packaged foods, always check the labels. Choose goods with as little artificial additives, preservatives, and added sugars as possible.

Setting up your South Beach kitchen is the first step to making healthy eating easy and enjoyable. By stocking up on the right ingredients, equipping your kitchen with the necessary tools, and planning your meals thoughtfully, you'll be ready to embrace this diet and make it a permanent part of your life. With a little effort and some organization, the kitchen will become a place where healthy habits thrive.

CHAPTER 4
Lifestyle Strategies for Success

The South Beach Diet is about more than just what you eat; it's a complete lifestyle change. To truly see success, it's important to incorporate exercise, make smart choices when dining out, manage social situations, and build lasting healthy habits. This chapter will guide you through these key areas to help you stay on track and enjoy your weight loss journey.

Exercise Recommendations

Exercise is a crucial part of maintaining overall health and supporting your weight loss goals on the South Beach Diet. While the diet focuses heavily on food choices, adding regular physical activity to your routine will speed up your progress, improve your energy levels, and enhance your overall well-being.

Why Exercise Matters

Exercise doesn't just help you burn calories—it also improves your cardiovascular health, strengthens muscles and bones, boosts metabolism, and reduces stress. The South Beach Diet emphasizes a balanced approach, and adding exercise ensures you're taking care of both your body and mind.

Getting Started

If you're new to exercise, start slow. Begin with simple activities and gradually increase the intensity and duration as your body adapts. To begin, you don't need expensive equipment or a gym membership. Consider the following kinds of exercise:

Cardio: Activities like walking, jogging, swimming, or cycling are excellent for increasing heart rate and burning fat. Aim for 30 minutes a day, five days a week, for the best results. You can break it up into shorter sessions if necessary, such as three 10-minute walks throughout the day.

Strength Training: Building muscle through strength training is essential, as muscle burns more calories at rest than fat. Simple exercises like squats, lunges, push-ups, or using resistance bands can be done at home. Every week, try to get in two or three strength training sessions.

Flexibility and Balance: Activities such as yoga, Pilates, or even stretching exercises help improve flexibility, reduce injury risk, and enhance overall body strength. Incorporating these activities can promote relaxation and mental clarity.

Creating a Routine

To stick to exercise, create a schedule that works for you. Every week, try to get in two or three strength training sessions. You don't need to spend hours at the gym—short, effective workouts can make a big difference.

To get you started, here is an example of a weekly routine:

Monday: 30 minute brisk walk + 15-minute full-body strength workout.

Tuesday: Yoga or Pilates for 30 minutes.
Wednesday: 30-minute walk or jog.
Thursday: 15-minute bodyweight strength workout.
Friday: 30-minute brisk walk.
Saturday: Yoga or stretching for 20 minutes.
Sunday: Rest or little exercise, as a leisurely stroll.

Finding Motivation
Maintain motivation by establishing reasonable objectives and monitoring your advancement. Whether it's increasing your walking time or adding more weight to your strength training, small improvements will keep you going. Don't forget to celebrate your milestones!

Eating Out Guidelines
One of the biggest challenges while following the South Beach Diet is eating out. Restaurants often serve foods that are high in unhealthy fats, sugars, and processed ingredients. However, with a little preparation and knowledge, you can stick to your goals even when dining out.

Know What to Order
The South Beach Diet encourages eating lean proteins, non-starchy vegetables, and healthy fats. Look for these options when ordering at restaurants:

Protein: Opt for grilled, baked, or steamed fish, chicken, turkey, or lean cuts of beef. Avoid anything fried or breaded.
Vegetables: Choose salads, grilled vegetables, or roasted vegetables as sides. Avoid starchy options like potatoes or pasta.

Healthy Fats: Ask for olive oil or avocado to be added to salads or dishes, and skip the creamy dressings or sauces.

Many restaurants offer healthy alternatives or will accommodate special requests, so don't be afraid to ask for modifications. For example, ask for your dressing on the side, request grilled meat instead of fried, or substitute vegetables for potatoes.

Portion Control

Restaurant portions tend to be larger than necessary, so consider asking for a to-go box when your meal is served. This way, you can enjoy half of your meal now and save the rest for later. Another trick is to order a starter-sized portion or share a main course with a friend.

Avoiding Temptation

When dining out, it's easy to give in to tempting, high-calorie foods. Stick to your goals by avoiding sugary cocktails, bread baskets, and high-calorie appetizers. If you're craving dessert, share a small portion with someone or opt for fresh fruit.

Smart Fast Food Choices

Fast food doesn't have to derail your diet. Many fast food chains now offer healthier options, such as grilled chicken salads or wraps. You can also ask for modifications like dressing on the side, no mayo, or extra vegetables. Be mindful of portion sizes and avoid high-calorie sides.

Handling Social Situations

Social situations, like family gatherings, parties, or work events, can present challenges when you're trying to follow the South Beach Diet. It's normal to feel tempted by foods that don't align with your goals, but with some preparation and confidence, you can navigate these events without straying from your plan.

Plan Ahead
If you know you'll be attending a social event, plan ahead by having a healthy snack or meal before you go. This way, you won't arrive hungry and tempted by unhealthy options. You can also bring your own dish to share, ensuring there's at least one South Beach-friendly option available.

Be Mindful at Buffets and Parties
Buffets and parties often feature a wide range of foods, many of which are high in carbs and fats. At a buffet, take a small plate and fill it with lean proteins and vegetables. Avoid the bread, chips, and sugary desserts. If you're at a party, don't hesitate to politely decline offers for non-South Beach-friendly foods, and focus on enjoying the social aspect of the event rather than the food.

Dealing with Pressure
Family and friends may not always understand why you're making healthier choices, and you might feel pressured to indulge. Be firm in your decision, and don't be afraid to explain that you're making changes for your health. Most people will respect your choice once they understand your commitment.

Navigating Alcohol

Alcohol can be a tricky part of social situations. While the South Beach Diet allows for moderate alcohol consumption in Phase 2 and Phase 3, it's important to be mindful of your choices. Opt for wine, light beer, or spirits mixed with soda water or a splash of juice. Avoid sugary cocktails, which can derail your progress.

Building Healthy Habits

Long-term success on the South Beach Diet isn't just about following the plan for a few weeks—it's about making lasting lifestyle changes. Building healthy habits that you can stick to for the long haul is the key to maintaining your weight loss and improving your overall health.

Start Small

It's easy to feel overwhelmed when making a big change, so start with small, manageable habits. Instead of overhauling everything at once, focus on one or two changes at a time. For example, start by cutting out sugary drinks or incorporating more vegetables into your meals. Once these changes become routine, add more healthy habits to your life.

Create a Routine

Maintaining a regular daily schedule can assist you in staying on course. Plan your meals ahead of time, set a regular exercise schedule, and make time for self-care. Having a routine will make healthy choices feel like second nature, and you'll be less likely to slip into old habits.

Track Your Progress

Monitoring your development is a fantastic method to maintain motivation. Keep a food diary or use an app to log your meals, workouts, and feelings. This will help you stay accountable and spot any patterns that might be sabotaging your progress.

Stay Positive

Weight loss and lifestyle changes take time, and there will be challenges along the way. Stay positive and patient with yourself. Celebrate your successes, no matter how small, and remember that setbacks are part of the process. Focus on the progress you've made, rather than any temporary obstacles.

Seek Support

A strong support network can significantly impact your path. Whether it's a friend, family member, or online community, connecting with others who are on the same path can provide motivation and encouragement. Share your successes, ask for advice, and offer support to others who are also striving for better health.

Incorporating exercise, making smart food choices when dining out, managing social situations, and building lasting healthy habits are all essential strategies for long-term success on the South Beach Diet. By adopting these lifestyle changes, you'll not only lose weight but also improve your overall well-being and build a sustainable, healthy lifestyle that will last for years to come. Remain consistent, stay focused, and relish the ride.

PART TWO: THE RECIPES

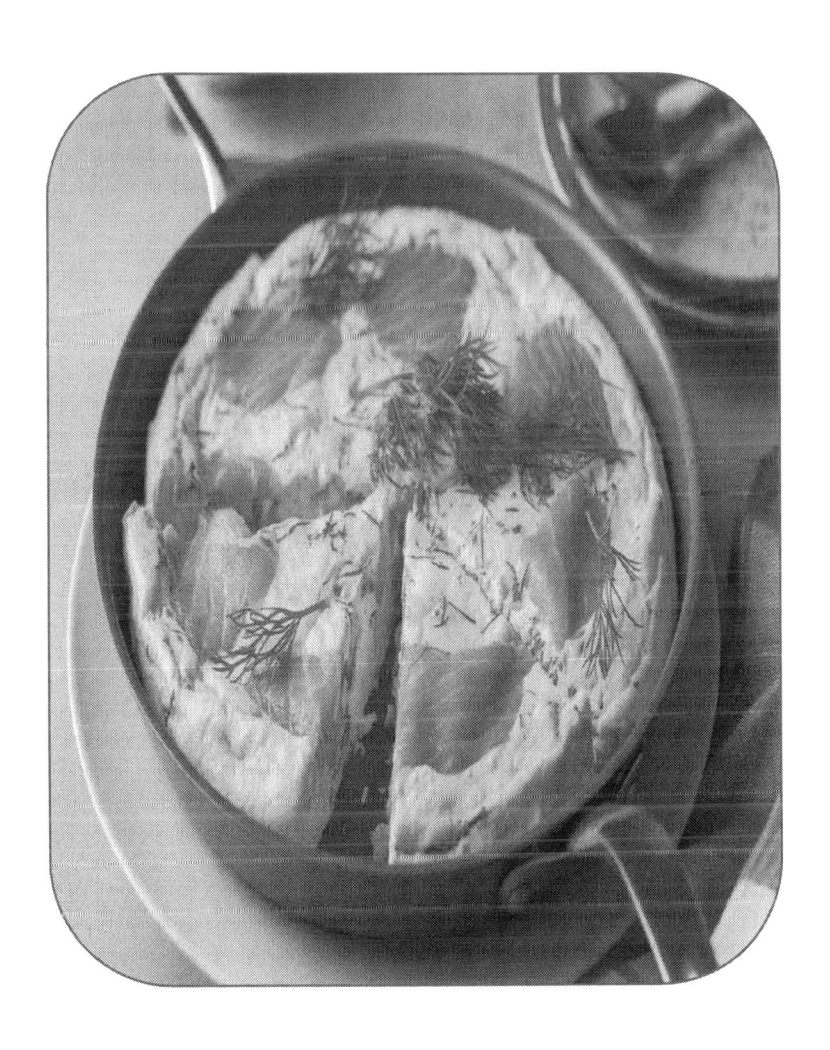

CHAPTER 5
Phase 1 Recipes (Two Week Reset)

Breakfast Recipes

Mediterranean Spinach and Feta Egg Cups

COOKING TIME: 20 MINUTES

SERVINGS: 4

Ingredients:
- 6 large eggs
- 1 cup fresh spinach, chopped
- 1/4 cup crumbled feta cheese
- 1 tablespoon olive oil
- Salt and pepper to taste

Instructions:
- Preheat your oven to 350°F (175°C). Use non-stick spray or olive oil to grease a muffin tray.
- Heat a small pan over medium heat and sauté the spinach with olive oil until wilted, about 2-3 minutes.
- Whisk the eggs in a bowl and add salt and pepper to taste.
- Stir up the feta cheese and sautéed spinach with the egg mixture.
- Evenly fill the muffin tin cups with the egg mixture.
- The eggs should be set and have a hint of golden color on top after fifteen to eighteen minutes of baking.
- Before serving, let it cool for couple of minutes.

Smoked Salmon and Dill Frittata

COOKING TIME: 25 MINUTES

SERVINGS: 4

Ingredients:
- 6 large eggs
- 1/2 cup smoked salmon, chopped
- 1/4 cup fresh dill, chopped
- 1/4 cup red onion, thinly sliced
- 1 tablespoon olive oil
- Salt and pepper to taste

Instructions:
- Preheat your oven to 375°F (190°C).
- Olive oil should be heated over a moderate flame in a medium ovenproof saucepan. Add the red onion and sauté for 2-3 minutes until soft.
- Add salt and pepper to the eggs after whisking them in a bowl.
- Add the smoked salmon and dill to the egg mixture and stir to combine.
- Pour the egg mixture into the skillet, making sure it evenly covers the onions.
- Cook for 5 minutes, then transfer the skillet to the oven and bake for 10-12 minutes, until the eggs are set.
- Before cutting into slices and serving, let it cool for a few minutes.

Turkey-Sage Breakfast Sausage with Roasted Peppers

COOKING TIME: 20 MINUTES

SERVINGS: 4

Ingredients:
- 1 lb ground turkey
- 1/2 teaspoon dried sage
- 1/4 teaspoon garlic powder
- 1/4 teaspoon onion powder
- 1 tablespoon olive oil
- 1 red bell pepper, chopped
- 1 yellow bell pepper, chopped
- Salt and pepper to taste

Instructions:
- In a bowl, combine the ground turkey, sage, garlic powder, onion powder, salt, and pepper. Mix well.
- Make tiny patties out of the turkey mixture that are two to three inches across.
- Add olive oil to a skillet and heat it over a moderate flame.
- The turkey patties should be cooked through and browned after four to five minutes on both sides in the saucepan.
- While the sausages are cooking, heat another skillet over medium heat and sauté the chopped bell peppers in a little olive oil for 5-6 minutes, until tender.
- Serve the turkey sausages with roasted peppers on the side.

Mexican-Style Cauliflower Rice Bowl with Eggs

COOKING TIME: 25 MINUTES

SERVINGS: 2

Ingredients:

2 large eggs
- 1 cup cauliflower rice (fresh or frozen)
- 1/2 cup diced tomatoes
- 1/4 cup onion, diced
- 1/4 teaspoon cumin
- 1/4 teaspoon chili powder
- 1 tablespoon olive oil
- Salt and pepper to taste

Instructions:
- Over a moderate flame, warm the olive oil in a big saucepan. Now, add the diced onion and sauté for two to three minutes.
- After adding the cauliflower rice to the saucepan simmer it for five to six minutes, stirring now and then, until it starts to get tender.
- Stir in the diced tomatoes, cumin, chili powder, salt, and pepper, and cook for another 3 minutes.
- Cook the eggs in a different pan until they are scrambled, poached, or sunny-side up.
- Divide the cauliflower rice mixture between two bowls and top each with a cooked egg.

Protein-Packed Green Smoothie Bowl
COOKING TIME: 10 MINUTES
SERVINGS: 1

Ingredients:
- 1/2 cup unsweetened almond milk
- 1/4 cup plain Greek yogurt
- 1 scoop protein powder (vanilla or unflavored)
- 1/2 cup spinach
- 1/4 avocado
- 1 tablespoon chia seeds
- Ice cubes (optional)
- *Toppings: sliced almonds, chia seeds, or unsweetened coconut flakes*

Instructions:
- In a blender, combine the almond milk, Greek yogurt, protein powder, spinach, avocado, and chia seeds.
- Blend until smooth. Use ice cubes to achieve a thicker consistency, if you desire.
- Pour the smoothie into a bowl and top with sliced almonds, extra chia seeds, or unsweetened coconut flakes.
- Enjoy immediately.

Asparagus and Goat Cheese Omelet
COOKING TIME: 15 MINUTES
SERVINGS: 2

Ingredients:
- 4 large eggs
- 1/2 cup fresh asparagus, chopped
- 2 tablespoons goat cheese, crumbled
- 1 tablespoon olive oil
- Salt and pepper to taste

Instructions:
- In a saucepan over a moderate flame, heat the olive oil. Sauté the chopped asparagus for three to four minutes, or until it becomes soft.
- In a mixing container, whisk together all of the eggs and season with salt and pepper.
- Cover the asparagus in the saucepan with the egg mixture. Allow the eggs to set by cooking them for two to three minutes.
- Fold one side of the omelet over the other and sprinkle the goat cheese on the other half.
- Serve immediately.

Coconut Chia Pudding with Sugar-Free Vanilla
COOKING TIME: 5 MINUTES (PLUS 2 HOURS TO SET)

SERVINGS: 2

Ingredients:
- 1/2 cup coconut milk (canned, full-fat or light)
- 2 tablespoons chia seeds
- 1/2 teaspoon vanilla extract (sugar-free)
- Select your preferred sweetener, to taste (erythritol, monk fruit, or stevia).

Instructions:
- In a small bowl, whisk together the coconut milk, chia seeds, vanilla extract, and sweetener.
- To enable the chia seeds to soak the liquid and develop a pudding-like consistency, cover and place in the refrigerator for at least two hours or overnight.
- Stir before serving, and enjoy chilled.

Zucchini-Herb Breakfast Pancakes (No Flour)
COOKING TIME: 15 MINUTES
SERVINGS: 4

Ingredients:
- 1 medium zucchini, grated
- 2 large eggs
- 1/4 teaspoon baking powder
- 1/4 teaspoon garlic powder
- 1 tablespoon fresh parsley, chopped
- Salt and pepper to taste
- 1 tablespoon olive oil for cooking

Instructions:
- Grate the zucchini and squeeze out excess water using a clean towel or paper towel.
- Add the grated zucchini, eggs, baking powder, parsley, garlic powder, salt, and pepper to a bowl.
- In a saucepan over a moderate flame, heat the olive oil.
- Create tiny pancakes by spooning the zucchini mixture into the griddle. Preheat the oven to between two and three minutes per side, or until golden brown.
- Serve immediately.

Buffalo Chicken Breakfast Muffins (Egg Base)

COOKING TIME: 25 MINUTES
SERVINGS: 6

Ingredients:
- 1 cup cooked chicken breast, shredded
- 6 large eggs
- 1/4 cup buffalo sauce (sugar-free)
- 1/4 cup shredded cheddar cheese (optional)
- Salt and pepper to taste

Instructions:
- Preheat your oven to 375°F (190°C). Grease a muffin tin with non-stick spray.
- Add salt and pepper to the eggs after whisking them in a bowl.
- Stir in the shredded chicken and buffalo sauce.
- Evenly distribute the egg and chicken mixture among the muffin tin cups.
- Top with shredded cheese, if desired.
- Bake for 15-20 minutes, or until the eggs are set and the muffins are lightly golden.
- Let cool for a few minutes before serving.

Mushroom and Swiss Breakfast Casserole

COOKING TIME: 30 MINUTES

SERVINGS: 4

Ingredients:

- 1 cup mushrooms, sliced
- 1/4 cup Swiss cheese, shredded
- 6 large eggs
- 1/4 cup unsweetened almond milk
- Salt and pepper to taste
- 1 tablespoon olive oil

Instructions:

- Preheat your oven to 350°F (175°C). Use non-stick spray or olive oil to grease a baking dish.
- Sauté the mushrooms in a saucepan over a moderate flame for five minutes, or until they are tender.
- Whisk the eggs and almond milk together in a mixing container and season with salt and pepper.
- Spread the sautéed mushrooms evenly in the baking dish and pour the egg mixture over them.
- Top with shredded Swiss cheese.
- Bake until the cheese is melted and bubbling and the eggs are set, between twenty and twenty-five minutes.
- After a few minutes of cooling, cut into slices and serve.

These Phase 1 breakfast recipes are designed to be simple, flavorful, and filling while helping you reset your body. Enjoy them as part of your two-week South Beach Diet journey!

Lunch Recipes

Thai-Style Lettuce Wraps with Ground Turkey

COOKING TIME: 20 MINUTES

SERVINGS: 4

Ingredients:
- 1 lb ground turkey
- 1 tablespoon olive oil
- 2 cloves garlic, minced
- 1 tablespoon fresh ginger, grated
- 2 tablespoons coconut aminos
- 1 tablespoon fish sauce
- 1 tablespoon lime juice
- 1 tablespoon sesame oil
- 1/2 cup shredded carrots
- 1/2 cup chopped cilantro
- 1/4 cup chopped green onions
- One head of iceberg lettuce or butter lettuce, with the leaves separated

Instructions:
- Over a moderate flame, warm the olive oil in a big saucepan. Add the ginger and garlic, and cook for about a minute, or until aromatic.
- Add the ground turkey and cook, breaking it up into crumbles, for 7-10 minutes until browned.
- Add fish sauce, lime juice, sesame oil, and coconut aminos and stir. To let the flavors, combine, cook for a further two minutes.
- Take off the heat and mix in the green onions, cilantro, and shredded carrots.

- Serve the turkey mixture by spooning it into the lettuce leaves.

Citrus-Poached Fish over Zucchini Noodles
COOKING TIME: 30 MINUTES
SERVINGS: 4

Ingredients:
- Four fillets of white fish, such tilapia or cod
- 2 cups low-sodium vegetable broth
- 1 orange, juiced
- 1 lemon, juiced
- 2 teaspoons lemon zest
- 2 tablespoons fresh parsley, chopped
- 2 zucchinis, spiralized into noodles
- 1 tablespoon olive oil
- Salt and pepper, to taste

Instructions:
- In a shallow pan, combine vegetable broth, orange juice, lemon juice, and lemon zest. Bring to a simmer over medium heat.
- Season the fish fillets with salt and pepper, then place them in the simmering broth. Poach the fish for 10 12 minutes until cooked through and easily flaked with a fork.
- While the fish is poaching, heat olive oil in a separate pan over medium heat. Add zucchini noodles and sauté for 3-5 minutes until tender. Season with salt and pepper.

- Place the poached fish on top of the zucchini noodles on a plate. Garnish with chopped parsley and serve.

Mediterranean Tuna and White Bean Salad

COOKING TIME: 15 MINUTES

SERVINGS: 4

Ingredients:
- Two cans (5 oz) of drained tuna in olive oil
- 15 ounces of washed and drained white beans from a can
- 1 cucumber, diced
- 1/2 red onion, finely chopped
- 1/2 cup cherry tomatoes, halved
- 1/4 cup Kalamata olives, pitted and chopped
- 2 tablespoons olive oil
- 1 tablespoon red wine vinegar
- 1 teaspoon dried oregano
- Salt and pepper, to taste

Instructions:
- In a large bowl, combine tuna, white beans, cucumber, red onion, tomatoes, and olives.
- Whisk together the oregano, red wine vinegar, olive oil, salt, and pepper in a small basin.
- Toss the salad to combine after adding the dressing.
- Serve right away or chill for half an hour to let the flavors combine.

Grilled Chicken Caesar Cloud Bread Sandwich

COOKING TIME: 30 MINUTES

SERVINGS: 4

Ingredients:
- 2 chicken breasts, grilled and sliced
- 4 cloud bread rounds (recipe below)
- 1/4 cup Caesar dressing (low-carb)
- 1/4 cup grated Parmesan cheese
- Freshly ground black pepper, to taste

Cloud Bread Ingredients:
- 3 large eggs, separated
- 3 oz cream cheese, softened
- 1/4 teaspoon cream of tartar
- 1/4 teaspoon baking powder
- 1/4 teaspoon sea salt

Instructions for Cloud Bread:
- Preheat your oven to 300°F (150°C). Line a baking sheet with parchment paper.
- Set aside the egg whites after beating them with the cream of tartar until stiff peaks form.
- In a separate bowl, blend egg yolks, cream cheese, baking powder, and salt until smooth.
- The egg whites should be gently folded into the yolk mixture until they are completely mixed.
- Spoon the mixture into rounds on the baking sheet and bake for 25-30 minutes until golden brown.
- Allow cloud bread to cool.

For the Sandwich:
- Spread Caesar dressing on the cloud bread rounds.
- Layer grilled chicken slices on top and sprinkle with Parmesan cheese and black pepper.
- Close the sandwich and serve.

Korean-Style Beef Bowl with Cauliflower Rice

COOKING TIME: 25 MINUTES

SERVINGS: 4

Ingredients:
- 1 lb ground beef
- 2 cloves garlic, minced
- 2 tablespoons coconut aminos
- 1 tablespoon sesame oil
- 1 tablespoon rice vinegar
- 1 teaspoon fresh ginger, grated
- 1 tablespoon honey (optional for sweetness)
- 4 cups cauliflower rice
- 1/4 cup green onions, chopped
- Sesame seeds, for garnish

Instructions:
- The sesame oil should be heated in a saucepan over a moderate flame. Cook for approximately one minute after adding the ginger and garlic.
- Break up the ground meat while it cooks and add it until it turns brown.
- Add rice vinegar, honey (if using), and coconut aminos and stir. Simmer for 3-5 minutes.
- Meanwhile, heat a separate pan and sauté cauliflower rice for 4-5 minutes until tender.
- Serve the beef over cauliflower rice, garnished with green onions and sesame seeds.

Shrimp and Avocado Stack with Citrus Dressing

COOKING TIME: 20 MINUTES

SERVINGS: 4

Ingredients:

- 1 lb shrimp, peeled and deveined
- 2 tablespoons olive oil
- 1 teaspoon paprika
- 1 avocado, diced
- 1/2 cucumber, diced
- 1/4 cup red onion, finely chopped
- 1 tablespoon lime juice
- 1 tablespoon orange juice
- 1 tablespoon olive oil
- Salt and pepper, to taste

Instructions:

- In a saucepan over a moderate flame, heat the olive oil. Add paprika, salt, and pepper to the shrimp before cooking them for two to three minutes on each side, or until they are opaque and pink.
- In a bowl, combine avocado, cucumber, red onion, lime juice, orange juice, and olive oil. Season with salt and pepper.
- Stack the shrimp on top of the avocado mixture and serve immediately.

Buffalo Chicken Stuffed Bell Peppers

COOKING TIME: 35 MINUTES

SERVINGS: 4

Ingredients:

- Four large bell peppers with the seeds removed and the tops cut off
- 2 cups cooked chicken breast, shredded
- 1/4 cup buffalo sauce (sugar-free)
- 1/4 cup cream cheese, softened
- 1/4 cup shredded cheddar cheese
- Salt and pepper, to taste

Instructions:

- Preheat the oven to 375°F (190°C).
- Put the cream cheese, shredded cheddar, buffalo sauce, and chicken shreds in a bowl. Season with salt and pepper.
- Fill bell peppers with buffalo chicken mixture.
- After placing them on a baking pan, bake the stuffed peppers for twenty-five to thirty minutes. or until they are soft.
- Serve hot.

Mediterranean Cauliflower Tabbouleh with Grilled Chicken

COOKING TIME: 20 MINUTES

SERVINGS: 4

Ingredients:

- 2 cups cauliflower rice, steamed
- 1 cucumber, diced
- 1/2 red onion, finely chopped
- 1/2 cup fresh parsley, chopped
- 1/4 cup fresh mint, chopped
- 2 tablespoons olive oil
- 1 tablespoon lemon juice
- Salt and pepper, to taste
- 2 grilled chicken breasts, sliced

Instructions:

- In a bowl, combine cauliflower rice, cucumber, red onion, parsley, and mint.
- After adding lemon juice and olive oil, season with salt and pepper. Toss to combine.
- Serve the tabbouleh with grilled chicken slices on top.

Asian-Inspired Salmon Power Bowl

COOKING TIME: 20 MINUTES
SERVINGS: 4

Ingredients:
- 4 salmon fillets
- 2 tablespoons sesame oil
- 1 tablespoon soy sauce (or coconut aminos)
- 1 tablespoon rice vinegar
- 1 teaspoon ginger, grated
- 1 cup spinach, sautéed
- 1/4 cup sliced cucumber
- 1/4 cup shredded carrots
- 1 tablespoon sesame seeds

Instructions:
- In a pan, heat the sesame oil over a moderate flame. Add salmon fillets and cook for 4-5 minutes on each side until cooked through.
- In a bowl, whisk together soy sauce, rice vinegar, and ginger.
- Serve the salmon over a bed of sautéed spinach, cucumber, and shredded carrots. Add sesame seeds as a garnish and drizzle with sauce.

Mexican Chicken Zucchini Boat

COOKING TIME: 30 MINUTES

SERVINGS: 4

Ingredients:
- 4 zucchinis, halved lengthwise and scooped out
- 2 cups cooked chicken breast, shredded
- 1/2 cup salsa (sugar-free)
- 1/2 cup shredded cheddar cheese
- 1 tablespoon olive oil
- Salt and pepper, to taste

Instructions:
- Preheat the oven to 375°F (190°C).
- Toss zucchini halves with olive oil, salt, and pepper. After placing it on a baking sheet, bake it for ten minutes.
- Mix shredded chicken with salsa, then spoon into the zucchini boats.
- Top with shredded cheddar cheese and bake for an additional 10-15 minutes until the cheese is melted and bubbly.
- Serve hot.

These lunch recipes are designed to help you stay on track with the South Beach Diet Phase 1 while enjoying delicious, healthy meals. Enjoy these tasty options as part of your two-week reset!

Approved Snacks

- Cucumber and Hummus
- Hard-Boiled Eggs with Salt and Pepper
- Crispy Roasted Chickpeas
- Celery Sticks with Almond Butter
- Sliced Turkey with Avocado
- Zucchini Chips
- Greek Yogurt with Berries
- Olives and Cheese
- Bell Pepper Slices with Guacamole
- Cottage Cheese with Sliced Tomatoes
- Roasted Almonds
- Carrot Sticks with Guacamole
- Baked Kale Chips
- Mini Caprese Salad (Mozzarella, Tomato, Basil)
- Smoked Salmon Rolls

14-Day Meal Plan

Here's a 14-day meal plan that follows the Phase 1 guidelines of the South Beach Diet. This meal plan includes a variety of simple and satisfying meals for breakfast, lunch, and dinner.

Day 1

Breakfast:
- Scrambled Eggs with Spinach and Feta Cheese

Quick, protein-packed, and filled with greens. Scramble 2 eggs and stir in a handful of spinach and some crumbled feta.

Lunch:

- Grilled Chicken Salad with Avocado and Olive Oil Dressing

Grilled chicken breast on a bed of mixed greens with slices of avocado, dressed with olive oil and lemon juice.

Dinner:
- Herb-Crusted Rack of Lamb with Roasted Vegetables

Season the lamb with rosemary, thyme, and garlic, roast with your choice of veggies like zucchini and bell peppers.

Day 2

Breakfast:
- Greek Yogurt with Berries

A simple, refreshing mix of plain Greek yogurt and a handful of fresh berries.

Lunch:
- Turkey-Stuffed Portobello Mushrooms

Hollow out Portobello mushrooms, stuff with lean ground turkey, herbs, and bake until golden.

Dinner:
- Blackened Fish with Cajun Cauliflower Rice

Blacken white fish like tilapia with Cajun spices, served with cauliflower rice sautéed with garlic.

Day 3

Breakfast:
- Cottage Cheese with Sliced Tomatoes

Enjoy fresh, creamy cottage cheese with sliced, ripe tomatoes and a sprinkle of salt and pepper.

Lunch:
- Zucchini Noodles with Pesto Chicken

Make zucchini noodles using a spiralizer, top with grilled chicken and homemade basil pesto.

Dinner:
- Coconut-Curry Chicken with Cauliflower Rice

Simmer chicken in coconut milk, curry paste, and spices, served with cauliflower rice for a creamy, satisfying dinner.

Day 4

Breakfast:
- Egg Muffins with Spinach and Cheese

Bake eggs in muffin tins with spinach, cheese, and a dash of salt and pepper for a portable breakfast.

Lunch:
- Grilled Shrimp Salad with Cucumber and Avocado

Grilled shrimp tossed in a fresh salad with cucumber, avocado, and a lemon-olive oil dressing.

Dinner:
- Grilled Steak with Chimichurri and Roasted Vegetables

Grill steak to your preference, topped with homemade chimichurri sauce, and serve with roasted veggies.

Day 5

Breakfast:
- Smoothie with Almond Milk, Spinach, and Protein Powder

Blend unsweetened almond milk with spinach, protein powder, and a handful of berries for a quick breakfast.

Lunch:
- Chicken Lettuce Wraps with Avocado

Cook chicken breast and slice thinly, then wrap in large lettuce leaves with avocado and a sprinkle of chili powder.

Dinner:
- Mediterranean Baked Cod with Olive Tapenade

Bake cod fillets with olive tapenade (chopped olives, capers, and olive oil), served with a side of roasted vegetables.

Day 6

Breakfast:
- Hard-Boiled Eggs with Salt and Pepper

A quick, no-fuss breakfast that's protein-rich and satisfying.

Lunch:
- Avocado Egg Salad

Mash avocado and boiled eggs together with lemon juice and season with salt and pepper for a creamy salad.

Dinner:
- Asian-Style Meatballs with Miracle Noodles

Ground chicken or turkey mixed with ginger and garlic, baked into meatballs and served with Miracle Noodles.

Day 7

Breakfast:
- Chia Pudding with Almond Milk and Berries

Soak chia seeds overnight in almond milk, and top with fresh berries in the morning.

Lunch:
- Turkey Lettuce Wraps with Mustard

Layer slices of turkey and mustard in a lettuce wrap for a low-carb lunch.

Dinner:
- Moroccan Spiced Chicken with Roasted Vegetables

Season chicken with Moroccan spices like cumin, coriander, and paprika, and roast with veggies like cauliflower and carrots.

Day 8

Breakfast:
- Scrambled Eggs with Avocado

Scramble eggs and serve with sliced avocado for a hearty, filling breakfast.

Lunch:

- Grilled Chicken with Kale and Lemon Dressing

Toss grilled chicken breast with fresh kale, a squeeze of lemon, and olive oil for a simple salad.

Dinner:
- Garlic Shrimp Scampi with Spaghetti Squash

Sauté shrimp in garlic butter and serve over roasted spaghetti squash for a light and satisfying dinner.

Day 9

Breakfast:

- Cottage Cheese with Sliced Cucumber

A simple, light breakfast of cottage cheese paired with crunchy cucumber slices.

Lunch:

- Spinach and Feta Stuffed Chicken Breast

Stuff chicken breasts with spinach and feta, bake, and serve with a side of roasted veggies.

Dinner:

- Herb-Crusted Pork Tenderloin with Mediterranean Vegetables

Coat pork tenderloin with a mixture of rosemary, thyme, and garlic, and serve with a Mediterranean vegetable mix.

Day 10

Breakfast:
- Egg Muffins with Bacon and Spinach

Bake eggs in muffin tins with crispy bacon and spinach for a savory, protein-rich breakfast.

Lunch:

- Zucchini and Turkey Stir Fry

Stir-fry zucchini and ground turkey with a dash of soy sauce for a light, savory lunch.

Dinner:

- Coconut-Curry Chicken with Cauliflower Rice

Recreate this delicious dinner from Day 3 for an easy-to-make, flavorful meal.

Day 11

Breakfast:
- Greek Yogurt with Almonds and Berries

Combine Greek yogurt with a handful of almonds and fresh berries for a balanced breakfast.

Lunch:
- Grilled Steak Salad with Avocado

Grilled steak slices tossed with fresh greens, avocado, and a balsamic vinaigrette.

Dinner:
- Blackened Fish with Cajun Cauliflower Rice

A repeat of Day 2's flavorful dinner, featuring Cajun-spiced fish and cauliflower rice.

Day 12

Breakfast:
- Chia Pudding with Almond Milk and Cinnamon

Soak chia seeds in almond milk, adding a sprinkle of cinnamon for added flavor.

Lunch:
- Chicken and Vegetable Stir Fry

Stir-fry chicken breast with bell peppers, onions, and zucchini for a simple, healthy lunch.

Dinner:

- Mediterranean Baked Cod with Olive Tapenade

Enjoy this dish again with its combination of light fish and tangy olive tapenade.

Day 13

Breakfast:
- Scrambled Eggs with Mushrooms and Feta

Scramble eggs with sautéed mushrooms and crumbled feta cheese for a savory breakfast.

Lunch:
- Turkey-Stuffed Portobello Mushrooms

A repeat of Day 2's lunch, stuffed with lean turkey and baked until golden.

Dinner:
- Grilled Steak with Chimichurri and Roasted Vegetables

Enjoy this juicy steak and flavorful chimichurri sauce again with your favorite roasted vegetables.

Day 14

Breakfast:
- Smoothie with Almond Milk and Spinach

Blend almond milk, spinach, and a scoop of protein powder for a nutrient-packed breakfast.

Lunch:
- Grilled Chicken Salad with Avocado

Enjoy this fresh and simple salad again with a few extra toppings like cucumber or olives.

Dinner:
- Garlic Shrimp Scampi with Spaghetti Squash

Recreate this satisfying dinner from Day 8, with juicy shrimp and light spaghetti squash.

This 14-day meal plan offers a wide variety of delicious, easy-to-make meals that will keep you satisfied and help you achieve your weight loss goals during the Phase 1 reset. Enjoy the meals and stay committed to your healthy eating journey!

CHAPTER 6
Phase 2 Recipes (Steady Loss)
Breakfast Recipes

Quinoa Breakfast Bowl with Berries and Almonds
COOKING TIME: 15 MINUTES
SERVINGS: 2

Ingredients:
- 1 cup quinoa
- 2 cups water or unsweetened almond milk
- 1/2 cup mixed berries (blueberries, raspberries, or strawberries)
- 1/4 cup sliced almonds
- 1 tablespoon chia seeds (optional)
- 1 tablespoon honey (optional)
- A pinch of cinnamon (optional)

Instructions:
- To get rid of its natural covering, rinse the quinoa under cold water.
- Heat the water (or almond milk) in a medium pot until it boils.
- Once the quinoa is in the saucepan, lower the heat to low, cover, and simmer for twelve to fifteen minutes, or until the quinoa is soft and the liquid has been absorbed.
- Fluff the quinoa with a fork and let it cool for a minute or two.

- Spoon the quinoa into bowls, then top with fresh berries, sliced almonds, chia seeds, and a drizzle of honey, if desired.
- Sprinkle a pinch of cinnamon on top for extra flavor, and serve.

Poached Eggs and Avocado on Whole Grain Toast

COOKING TIME: 10 MINUTES

SERVINGS: 2

Ingredients:
- 2 slices of whole grain bread
- 1 ripe avocado
- 4 large eggs
- 1 tablespoon white vinegar (for poaching)
- Salt and pepper, to taste
- Optional: chili flakes for extra flavor

Instructions:
- Toast the slices of whole grain bread in a toaster or on a grill pan until golden and crispy.
- Make a kettle of water simmer gently while the bread toasts. Add the vinegar to the water.
- Gently transfer the cracked eggs into little cups into the water that is simmering. Eggs should be poached for three to four minutes if you want runny yolks, or longer if you want firmer yolks.
- In a bowl, mash the avocado and add salt and pepper while the eggs are cooking.
- Once the toast is ready, spread the mashed avocado evenly over each slice of bread.
- Using a slotted spoon, remove the poached eggs from the water and place them on top of the avocado toast.
- If preferred, add more chili flakes, salt, and pepper for seasoning. Serve immediately.

Steel-Cut Oats with Cinnamon Apple and Walnuts
COOKING TIME: 25 MINUTES
SERVINGS: 2

Ingredients:
- 1 cup steel-cut oats
- 3 cups water or unsweetened almond milk
- 1 medium apple, diced
- 1/4 cup chopped walnuts
- 1 teaspoon ground cinnamon
- 1 teaspoon vanilla extract (optional)
- 1 tablespoon honey or maple syrup (optional)

Instructions:
- Heat the water or almond milk in a medium-size saucepan until it boils.
- Add the steel-cut oats, reduce the heat to low, and simmer uncovered for 20-25 minutes, stirring occasionally until the oats are tender and creamy.
- A small saucepan should be heated to medium heat while the oats are cooking. Add the diced apple and cook for about 5 minutes until soft. Sprinkle with cinnamon.
- Once the oats are ready, stir in the vanilla extract, if using.
- Spoon the oats into bowls, and top with the cinnamon apples, chopped walnuts, and a drizzle of honey or maple syrup.
- Serve warm and enjoy.

Greek Yogurt Parfait with Homemade Sugar-Free Granola

COOKING TIME: 5 MINUTES (GRANOLA PREPARATION NOT INCLUDED)

SERVINGS: 2

Ingredients:
- 1 cup plain Greek yogurt
- 1/2 cup homemade sugar-free granola (or store-bought, if preferred)
- 1/4 cup mixed berries (blueberries, strawberries)
- 1 tablespoon chia seeds (optional)
- 1 teaspoon honey (optional)

Instructions:
- In two glasses or bowls, layer the Greek yogurt on the bottom.
- Add a layer of homemade sugar-free granola on top of the yogurt.
- Layer the mixed berries and sprinkle with chia seeds, if using.
- Drizzle with honey for sweetness, if desired.
- Repeat the layers and finish with a final topping of granola and berries.
- Serve immediately, or refrigerate for later.

Buckwheat Pancakes with Mixed Berry Compote

COOKING TIME: 20 MINUTES

SERVINGS: 4 PANCAKES (2 SERVINGS)

Ingredients:
- 1 cup buckwheat flour
- 1 tablespoon baking powder
- 1/4 teaspoon salt
- 1 egg
- 3/4 cup unsweetened almond milk
- 1 teaspoon vanilla extract
- 1 cup mixed berries (for the compote)
- 1 tablespoon honey (for the compote)
- 1 tablespoon water (for the compote)

Instructions:
- Add the baking powder, salt, and buckwheat flour to a large bowl.
- Whisk the egg, almond milk, and vanilla extract in another bowl.
- Stir just until mixed after adding the wet components to the dry ingredients. The batter should be thick but pourable.
- Apply cooking spray or oil to a non-stick skillet or griddle and heat it over medium heat.
- For each pancake, add roughly a quarter cup of batter to the saucepan. Cook until golden brown, about two or three minutes per side.
- While the pancakes are cooking, make the compote. In a small saucepan, combine the mixed berries, honey, and water. Simmer over low heat for 5-7 minutes until

the berries release their juices and form a syrupy compote.
- Top the pancakes with the berry compote and serve them warm.

Sweet Potato and Turkey Breakfast Hash

COOKING TIME: 20 MINUTES

SERVINGS: 2

Ingredients:
- 1 medium sweet potato, peeled and diced
- 1 tablespoon olive oil
- 1/2 onion, chopped
- 1/2 red bell pepper, chopped
- 1/2-pound ground turkey
- Salt and pepper, to taste
- 1 teaspoon smoked paprika (optional)
- 2 eggs (optional, for serving)

Instructions:
- Over a moderate flame, warm the olive oil in a big saucepan.
- Add the diced sweet potato to the skillet and cook for 8-10 minutes, stirring occasionally, until they begin to soften.
- Cook the diced onions and red bell pepper in the saucepan for a further five minutes, or until they are soft.

- In a separate pan, cook the ground turkey over medium heat, breaking it apart with a spoon. Season with salt, pepper, and smoked paprika.
- When the turkey is done, put it in the saucepan with the sweet potato mixture and mix everything together.
- If desired, place a properly fried or poached egg on the top.
- Serve immediately, and enjoy a filling and nutritious breakfast.

Whole Grain English Muffin with Egg and Spinach

COOKING TIME: 10 MINUTES

SERVINGS: 1

Ingredients:
- 1 whole grain English muffin, halved
- 1 large egg
- 1/2 cup spinach, sautéed
- Salt and pepper, to taste
- 1 tablespoon olive oil (for sautéing spinach)

Instructions:
- Toast the English muffin halves until golden.
- While the muffin is toasting, heat the olive oil in a small skillet over medium heat. Sauté the spinach for two to three minutes, or until it wilts.
- In another pan, cook the egg to your liking (fried, scrambled, or poached).
- After the egg has been cooked, place the sautéed spinach on one side of the muffin.
- Season with salt and pepper, then serve immediately.

Overnight Chia-Oat Pudding with Peaches
COOKING TIME: 5 MINUTES (OVERNIGHT REST)

SERVINGS: 2

Ingredients:
- 1/4 cup rolled oats
- 2 tablespoons chia seeds
- 3/4 cup unsweetened almond milk
- 1/2 teaspoon vanilla extract
- 1/2 peach, diced (or any fruit of choice)
- 1 teaspoon honey (optional)

Instructions:
- Put the almond milk, chia seeds, rolled oats, and vanilla essence in a bowl or container. Stir well.
- Cover and refrigerate overnight.
- In the morning, stir the mixture again, then top with fresh diced peaches and a drizzle of honey.
- Serve chilled, and enjoy your easy and nutritious breakfast.

Protein Power Toast with Ricotta and Figs

COOKING TIME: 10 MINUTES
SERVINGS: 1

Ingredients:
- 1 slice whole grain bread
- 1/4 cup ricotta cheese
- 2 fresh figs, sliced
- 1 teaspoon honey
- A pinch of cinnamon (optional)

Instructions:
- To achieve the necessary level of crispness, toast the whole grain bread.
- Spread the ricotta cheese evenly over the toast.
- Top with the chopped figs and pour honey over them.
- Optionally, sprinkle with cinnamon for extra flavor.
- Serve immediately for a delicious and protein-packed breakfast.

Brown Rice Breakfast Porridge with Nuts

COOKING TIME: 20 MINUTES

SERVINGS: 2

Ingredients:
- 1 cup cooked brown rice
- 1 1/2 cups unsweetened almond milk
- 1 tablespoon chia seeds
- 1/4 cup mixed nuts (almonds, walnuts, cashews)
- 1 tablespoon honey or maple syrup (optional)

Instructions:
- Almond milk and cooked brown rice should be combined in a medium-sized saucepan. Heat over medium heat until warmed through.
- Stir in the chia seeds and let the mixture simmer for 5-7 minutes, stirring occasionally.
- Once the porridge thickens, spoon it into bowls.
- Top with mixed nuts and a drizzle of honey or maple syrup, if desired.
- Serve warm and enjoy a comforting, wholesome breakfast.

These breakfast recipes are perfect for Phase 2 of the South Beach Diet, combining healthy ingredients with great taste to keep you satisfied as you continue your journey toward steady weight loss.

Lunch Recipes

Quinoa Buddha Bowl with Grilled Chicken

COOKING TIME: 25 MINUTES

SERVINGS: 2

Ingredients:
- 1 cup quinoa
- 2 chicken breasts
- 1 tablespoon olive oil
- 1 teaspoon paprika
- 1 teaspoon garlic powder
- Salt and pepper to taste
- 1 cup mixed greens (spinach, arugula)
- 1/2 cucumber, sliced
- 1/2 cup cherry tomatoes, halved
- 1/4 cup shredded carrots
- 1/4 cup hummus (optional)

Instructions:
- Rinse the quinoa under cold water. Put the quinoa and two cups of water in a saucepan. Bring it to a boil, reduce heat, and let it simmer for 15-20 minutes until the water is absorbed and the quinoa is tender.
- While the quinoa is cooking, season the chicken breasts with olive oil, paprika, garlic powder, salt, and pepper.
- Grill the chicken breasts on medium heat for 5-7 minutes per side or until fully cooked. Before slicing, let them a few minutes to rest.

- The cooked quinoa should be spread out in two bowls. Add shredded carrots, cherry tomatoes, cucumber slices, and mixed greens on top.
- After grilling, cut the chicken into slices and place it over the vegetables.
- Serve with a dollop of hummus, if desired.

Mediterranean Chickpea and Tuna Salad

COOKING TIME: 10 MINUTES

SERVINGS: 2

Ingredients:
- 1 can chickpeas, drained and rinsed
- 1 can tuna in water, drained
- 1/2 cucumber, chopped
- 1/2 red onion, finely chopped
- 1/4 cup Kalamata olives, sliced
- 1/4 cup feta cheese, crumbled
- 1 tablespoon olive oil
- 1 tablespoon lemon juice
- Salt and pepper to taste
- 1 teaspoon dried oregano

Instructions:
- In a large bowl, combine chickpeas, tuna, cucumber, red onion, olives, and feta cheese.
- Olive oil and lemon juice should be drizzled over the items.
- Season with salt, pepper, and oregano.

- Toss everything together until well mixed. Serve immediately or refrigerate for later.

Whole Grain Tortilla Wrap with Turkey and Avocado

COOKING TIME: 10 MINUTES

SERVINGS: 2

Ingredients:
- 4 slices turkey breast (preferably lean)
- 1 ripe avocado, sliced
- 1 tablespoon mustard or hummus (optional)
- 2 whole grain tortillas
- 1/4 cup spinach leaves
- Salt and pepper to taste

Instructions:
- On a spotless surface, spread the whole grain tortillas out flat.
- Spread mustard or hummus on each tortilla (optional).
- Layer the turkey slices, avocado, and spinach on the tortillas.
- Season with salt and pepper.
- After securely rolling the tortillas, cut them in half.

Lentil and Grilled Vegetable Power Bowl
COOKING TIME: 30 MINUTES
SERVINGS: 2

Ingredients:
- 1 cup cooked lentils
- 1 zucchini, sliced
- 1 bell pepper, sliced
- 1 red onion, sliced
- 1 tablespoon olive oil
- 1 teaspoon dried basil
- 1 tablespoon balsamic vinegar
- Salt and pepper to taste

Instructions:
- Set the grill pan or grill over a moderate temperature.
- Combine the red onion, bell pepper, and zucchini with the olive oil, salt, pepper, and basil.
- Grill the vegetables for 5-7 minutes on each side until they are tender and have grill marks.
- In a bowl, combine the cooked lentils and grilled vegetables.
- Drizzle balsamic vinegar over the top and serve warm.

Asian-Inspired Brown Rice Bowl with Salmon

COOKING TIME: 25 MINUTES

SERVINGS: 2

Ingredients:
- 1 cup brown rice
- 2 salmon fillets
- 2 tablespoons soy sauce (low-sodium)
- 1 tablespoon sesame oil
- 1 teaspoon ginger, grated
- 1/2 cucumber, julienned
- 1/4 cup edamame beans (cooked)
- 1 tablespoon sesame seeds

Instructions:
- Cook the brown rice according to package instructions (usually takes about 20 minutes).
- Sesame oil should be heated in a saucepan over a moderate flame. After adding salt and pepper to taste, sauté the salmon fillets for four to five minutes on each side, or until they are cooked through and golden.
- In a small bowl, mix the soy sauce and grated ginger. Drizzle the mixture over the salmon during the last minute of cooking.
- Once the rice is ready, divide it between two bowls.
- Top with the grilled salmon, cucumber, edamame beans, and sesame seeds.
- Serve immediately.

Greek Chicken Pita with Whole Grain Bread

COOKING TIME: 20 MINUTES

SERVINGS: 2

Ingredients:
- 2 whole grain pita pockets
- 2 grilled chicken breasts, sliced
- 1/4 cup tzatziki sauce
- 1/2 cucumber, chopped
- 1/4 cup red onion, sliced thin
- 1/4 cup Kalamata olives, chopped
- Fresh parsley for garnish

Instructions:
- Slice the grilled chicken breasts into thin strips.
- Warm the whole grain pita pockets in a dry skillet or oven.
- Fill each pita with a dollop of tzatziki sauce.
- Place grilled chicken, red onion, cucumber, and olives inside the pitas.
- Garnish with fresh parsley and serve immediately.

Black Bean and Sweet Potato Burrito Bowl

COOKING TIME: 30 MINUTES

SERVINGS: 2

Ingredients:
- 1 large sweet potato, diced
- 1 can black beans, drained and rinsed
- 1 tablespoon olive oil
- 1 teaspoon chili powder
- 1/2 teaspoon cumin
- Salt and pepper to taste
- 1/2 cup corn kernels
- 1/2 avocado, sliced
- 1 tablespoon cilantro, chopped

Instructions:
- Preheat the oven to 400°F (200°C). Toss the diced sweet potato in olive oil, chili powder, cumin, salt, and pepper.
- Spread the sweet potato on a baking sheet and roast for 20-25 minutes, flipping halfway through, until tender.
- In a saucepan set over a moderate flame, cook the corn and black beans while the sweet potato roasts.
- Once the sweet potato is done, assemble the burrito bowl by layering the sweet potato, black beans, corn, avocado slices, and cilantro.
- Serve warm.

Farro Salad with Grilled Shrimp

COOKING TIME: 25 MINUTES

SERVINGS: 2

Ingredients:
- 1 cup farro, cooked
- 1/2-pound shrimp, peeled and deveined
- 1 tablespoon olive oil
- 1 teaspoon garlic powder
- Salt and pepper to taste
- 1/4 cup cherry tomatoes, halved
- 1/4 cup cucumber, chopped
- 1 tablespoon lemon juice
- Fresh parsley for garnish

Instructions:
- Cook the farro according to the package directions (about 20 minutes).
- Set an outside grill or grill pan over a moderate temperature.
- Toss the shrimp in olive oil, garlic powder, salt, and pepper.
- The shrimp should be pink and opaque after two to three minutes on each side of the grill.
- In a bowl, combine the cooked farro, grilled shrimp, cherry tomatoes, cucumber, and lemon juice.
- Garnish with fresh parsley and serve.

Turkey Club on Ezekiel Bread
COOKING TIME: 15 MINUTES
SERVINGS: 2

Ingredients:
- 4 slices Ezekiel bread
- 4 slices turkey breast
- 2 slices tomato
- 2 leaves romaine lettuce
- 2 slices avocado
- 1 tablespoon mustard (optional)
- Salt and pepper to taste

Instructions:
- Toast the Ezekiel bread until golden.
- Spread mustard on one side of each slice of toast (optional).
- Layer the turkey, tomato slices, lettuce, and avocado on two slices of bread.
- Season with salt and pepper.
- Cut the bread in half, place the remaining pieces on top, and serve.

Mason Jar Chickpea and Quinoa Salad
COOKING TIME: 10 MINUTES

SERVINGS: 2

Ingredients:
- 1/2 cup cooked quinoa
- 1/2 cup chickpeas, drained and rinsed
- 1/4 cup cucumber, diced
- 1/4 cup cherry tomatoes, halved
- 1 tablespoon olive oil
- 1 tablespoon lemon juice
- Salt and pepper to taste
- 1 tablespoon fresh parsley, chopped

Instructions:
- In a mason jar, layer the ingredients starting with quinoa, followed by chickpeas, cucumber, and cherry tomatoes.
- Drizzle with olive oil and lemon juice.
- Season with salt, pepper, and fresh parsley.
- Close the jar and shake before serving. Enjoy a quick and fresh salad!

These lunch recipes are designed for Phase 2 of the South Beach Diet, focusing on balanced meals that will keep you full and energized throughout the day. Each dish is packed with nutrient-dense ingredients and is easy to prepare. Enjoy!

Dinner Recipes

Grilled Fish with Ancient Grain Pilaf

COOKING TIME: 30 MINUTES

SERVINGS: 2

Ingredients:
- 2 fish fillets (salmon, tilapia, or cod)
- 1 tablespoon olive oil
- 1 lemon, sliced
- 1 teaspoon garlic powder
- Salt and pepper to taste
- 1 cup ancient grains (quinoa, farro, or millet)
- 2 cups vegetable broth or water
- 1/4 cup chopped parsley

Instructions:
- Set the grill pan or grill over a moderate temperature to preheat.
- Drizzle olive oil over the fish fillets and season with garlic powder, salt, and pepper.
- The fish should be cooked through after grilling for four to five minutes on each side. Add lemon slices to the grill for extra flavor.
- In a saucepan, combine the ancient grains with vegetable broth or water. Bring to a boil, then lower the heat and simmer until the grains are soft, approximately twenty minutes.
- Using a fork, fluff the grains and mix in the chopped parsley.

- Serve the grilled fish on top of the ancient grain pilaf with the grilled lemon slices for added flavor.

Turkey Meatballs with Whole Wheat Pasta
COOKING TIME: 40 MINUTES
SERVINGS: 4

Ingredients:
- 1-pound ground turkey
- 1/4 cup grated Parmesan cheese
- 1/4 cup breadcrumbs (whole wheat)
- 1 egg
- 2 cloves garlic, minced
- 1 teaspoon dried oregano
- Salt and pepper to taste
- 3 cups marinara sauce (low-sugar)
- 8 ounces whole wheat pasta

Instructions:
- Preheat the oven to 375°F (190°C).
- In a bowl, combine ground turkey, Parmesan, breadcrumbs, egg, garlic, oregano, salt, and pepper.
- Put the mixture on a baking sheet and shape it into meatballs that are approximately one inch in diameter.
- The meatballs should be cooked through after twenty to twenty-five minutes in the oven.
- Prepare the whole wheat pasta as directed on the package while the meatballs are baking.

- In a large saucepan cook the marinara sauce over a moderate flame. Simmer for five to ten minutes after adding the roasted meatballs to the sauce.
- Serve the turkey meatballs over the cooked whole wheat pasta, garnished with extra Parmesan if desired.

Chicken and Brown Rice Stir-Fry
COOKING TIME: 30 MINUTES
SERVINGS: 4

Ingredients:
- 2 chicken breasts, diced
- 1 cup cooked brown rice
- 1 tablespoon olive oil
- 1/2 onion, sliced
- 1 bell pepper, sliced
- 1 carrot, julienned
- 2 cloves garlic, minced
- 2 tablespoons soy sauce (low-sodium)
- 1 tablespoon sesame oil
- 1 tablespoon rice vinegar
- Salt and pepper to taste

Instructions:
- In a big wok or saucepan heat the olive oil over a moderate flame.
- Add diced chicken breasts and cook for 5-7 minutes, or until browned and cooked through. Remove from the skillet and set aside.

- In the same skillet, add onion, bell pepper, carrot, and garlic. For three to five minutes, stir-fry the vegetables until they start to soften.
- Put the rice vinegar, sesame oil, soy sauce, and cooked brown rice in the saucepan. Stir well to combine.
- Put the chicken back in the saucepan and combine all the ingredients. Cook for an additional 2-3 minutes.
- Season with salt and pepper to taste. Serve hot.

Black Bean and Quinoa Stuffed Bell Peppers

COOKING TIME: 40 MINUTES
SERVINGS: 2

Ingredients:
- 2 large bell peppers, halved and seeds removed
- 1 cup cooked quinoa
- 1 can black beans, drained and rinsed
- 1/2 cup diced tomatoes
- 1 teaspoon cumin
- 1/2 teaspoon chili powder
- Salt and pepper to taste
- 1/4 cup shredded cheese (optional)

Instructions:
- Preheat the oven to 375°F (190°C).
- Place the bell pepper halves on a baking sheet and roast for 15 minutes.
- Combine your cooked quinoa, black beans, chopped tomatoes, chili powder, cumin, salt, and pepper in a mixing bowl.

- Top the stuffed peppers with some shredded cheese, if you'll be us
- Remove the bell peppers from the oven and stuff them with the quinoa mixture.ing.
- To ensure the peppers are soft and the cheese is melted, put the stuffed peppers back in the oven and bake them for a further fifteen to twenty minutes.
- Serve hot.

Mediterranean Lamb with Couscous
COOKING TIME: 35 MINUTES
SERVINGS: 2

Ingredients:
- 2 lamb chops
- 1 tablespoon olive oil
- 1 teaspoon dried rosemary
- 1 teaspoon garlic powder
- Salt and pepper to taste
- 1 cup couscous
- 1 1/4 cups vegetable broth
- 1/4 cup chopped cucumber
- 1/4 cup cherry tomatoes, halved
- 2 tablespoons fresh parsley, chopped

Instructions:
- Set the grill pan or grill over a moderate flame to preheat.

- Sprinkle salt, pepper, garlic powder, and rosemary over the lamb chops after drizzling them with olive oil.
- Grill the lamb chops for 4-5 minutes on each side for medium-rare, or cook to your preferred doneness.
- While the lamb is cooking, prepare the couscous. Heat the veggie broth in a saucepan until it boils. Reduce the heat, add the couscous, and cover. After five minutes, use a fork to fluff it.
- In a bowl, mix together cucumber, cherry tomatoes, and parsley.
- Serve the grilled lamb chops on a bed of couscous and top with the cucumber-tomato mixture.

Herb-Crusted Salmon with Wild Rice

COOKING TIME: 30 MINUTES

SERVINGS: 2

Ingredients:
- 2 salmon fillets
- 1 tablespoon olive oil
- 1 teaspoon dried thyme
- 1 teaspoon dried dill
- Salt and pepper to taste
- 1 cup wild rice
- 2 cups vegetable broth
- 1 tablespoon lemon juice

Instructions:
- Preheat the oven to 400°F (200°C).
- Place the salmon fillets on a baking sheet. Add salt, pepper, dill, and thyme to taste, then drizzle with olive oil.
- The salmon should be cooked through after twelve to fifteen minutes in the oven.
- Follow the directions on the package to boil the wild rice in vegetable stock while the salmon bakes.
- Once the rice is cooked, fluff it with a fork and stir in lemon juice.
- Serve the herb-crusted salmon over the wild rice.

Turkey and Sweet Potato Shepherd's Pie

COOKING TIME: 45 MINUTES

SERVINGS: 4

Ingredients:
- 1-pound ground turkey
- 2 large sweet potatoes, peeled and diced
- 1/2 cup low-sodium chicken broth
- 1/2 cup frozen peas
- 1/2 cup diced carrots
- 1 teaspoon dried thyme
- Salt and pepper to taste

Instructions:
- Preheat the oven to 375°F (190°C).
- In a large pan, cook ground turkey over medium heat until browned. Season with salt, pepper, and thyme.
- Add frozen peas and diced carrots to the pan and cook for 5 minutes.
- In a separate pot, boil the diced sweet potatoes in water until soft, about 10-15 minutes.
- Drain the sweet potatoes and mash them with chicken broth until smooth.
- Transfer the turkey mixture to a baking dish and spread the mashed sweet potatoes over the top.
- Bake until the top is just beginning to turn brown, around twenty minutes. Serve warm.

Shrimp and Whole Grain Pasta Primavera

COOKING TIME: 25 MINUTES

SERVINGS: 4

Ingredients:
- 1-pound shrimp, peeled and deveined
- 8 ounces whole grain pasta
- 1 tablespoon olive oil
- 1 zucchini, sliced
- 1 bell pepper, sliced
- 1/2 cup cherry tomatoes, halved
- 1/4 cup fresh basil, chopped
- 1 tablespoon lemon juice
- Salt and pepper to taste

Instructions:
- Follow the directions on the package to prepare the whole grain pasta.
- Over a moderate flame, warm the olive oil in a big saucepan.
- Add shrimp to the skillet and cook for 3-4 minutes per side, until pink and opaque. Remove the shrimp and set aside.
- Add the cherry tomatoes, bell pepper, and zucchini to the same saucepan. Cook the vegetables for about five to seven minutes, or until they are soft.
- Return the shrimp to the saucepan along with the cooked pasta. Stir to combine.
- Drizzle with lemon juice and season with salt and pepper. Garnish with fresh basil before serving.

Asian-Style Beef with Soba Noodles

COOKING TIME: 30 MINUTES

SERVINGS: 4

Ingredients:
- 1-pound flank steak, thinly sliced
- 8 ounces soba noodles
- 2 tablespoons soy sauce (low-sodium)
- 1 tablespoon sesame oil
- 2 teaspoons ginger, grated
- 2 cloves garlic, minced
- 1/2 cup sliced green onions
- 1/4 cup sesame seeds

Instructions:
- Cook soba noodles according to package instructions. Drain and set aside.
- Heat the sesame oil in a large saucepan over moderately high heat.
- Add the sliced beef and cook for 5-7 minutes, or until browned.
- Add garlic, ginger, soy sauce, and green onions. Cook for an additional 2-3 minutes.
- Toss the cooked soba noodles in the skillet and stir to combine.
- Garnish with sesame seeds before serving.

Baked Chicken with Quinoa and Roasted Vegetables

COOKING TIME: 45 MINUTES
SERVINGS: 4

Ingredients:
- 4 chicken breasts
- 1 tablespoon olive oil
- 1 teaspoon paprika
- 1 teaspoon garlic powder
- Salt and pepper to taste
- 1 cup cooked quinoa
- 2 cups mixed vegetables (carrots, broccoli, bell peppers)

Instructions:
- Preheat the oven to 400°F (200°C).
- Add salt, pepper, garlic powder, and paprika to the chicken breasts after drizzling them with olive oil.
- The chicken should be cooked through after about twenty-five to thirty minutes of baking on a baking sheet.
- Meanwhile, toss mixed vegetables in olive oil and season with salt and pepper. Roast in the oven for 15-20 minutes.
- Serve the baked chicken with quinoa and roasted vegetables on the side

Phase 2 of the South Beach Diet focuses on steady weight loss. During this phase, you can start to incorporate more healthy carbs, like whole grains, legumes, and fruits, while still keeping the focus on lean proteins, vegetables, and healthy fats. The idea is to maintain a balanced diet that keeps you feeling satisfied while losing weight steadily. This chapter includes recipes that fit within the Phase 2 guidelines, along with a 14-day meal plan to help you stay on track.

Approved Snacks

- Celery and Peanut Butter
- Greek Yogurt with Almonds
- Hard-Boiled Eggs
- Cottage Cheese with Cherry Tomatoes
- Apple with Almond Butter
- Carrot Sticks with Hummus
- Mixed Nuts (unsalted)
- Cucumber Slices with Guacamole
- Cheese Sticks (low-fat)
- Turkey or Chicken Roll-Ups
- Edamame Beans
- Chia Seed Pudding
- Sliced Bell Peppers with Salsa
- Roasted Chickpeas
- Avocado Slices with Lemon and Salt

14-Day Meal Plan

Here is a simple and healthy 14-day meal plan using the recipes from Chapter 6. This plan helps you stay on track for steady weight loss, offering a variety of meals that are delicious, nutritious, and satisfying.

Day 1

Breakfast
- **Scrambled Eggs with Spinach and Feta**

2 eggs scrambled with spinach, onions, and crumbled feta cheese.

Lunch
- **Grilled Chicken Salad with Avocado**

Grilled chicken, mixed greens, cucumber, cherry tomatoes, and avocado. Dress with olive oil and lemon juice.

Dinner
- **Baked Salmon with Steamed Broccoli and Quinoa**

A baked salmon fillet seasoned with lemon and herbs, served with steamed broccoli and cooked quinoa.

Day 2

Breakfast
- **Greek Yogurt with Fresh Berries and Walnuts**

A bowl of plain Greek yogurt topped with fresh blueberries, raspberries, and chopped walnuts.

Lunch
- **Turkey and Avocado Lettuce Wraps**

Slices of lean turkey and avocado are wrapped in big lettuce leaves. For added taste, throw some cheese over top.

Dinner
- **Grilled chicken and tomato sauce over zucchini noodles**

Zucchini noodles sautéed with olive oil and garlic, topped with homemade tomato sauce and grilled chicken.

Day 3

Breakfast
- **Veggie Omelet**

An omelet made with 2 eggs, bell peppers, onions, and spinach. Top with a small amount of shredded cheese.

Lunch
- **Shrimp and Avocado Salad**

Grilled shrimp with mixed greens, avocado, cucumber, and a lemon vinaigrette dressing.

Dinner
- **Turkey Meatballs with Roasted Cauliflower and Brussels Sprouts**

Baked turkey meatballs with roasted cauliflower and Brussels sprouts, drizzled with olive oil and balsamic vinegar.

Day 4

Breakfast
- **Chia Seed Pudding with Almonds and Strawberries**

Chia seeds soaked overnight in unsweetened almond milk, topped with fresh strawberries and sliced almonds.

Lunch
- **Grilled Chicken and Veggie Skewers**

Chicken skewers with zucchini, bell peppers, and onions, grilled and served with a side of Greek yogurt dipping sauce.

Dinner
- *Baked Chicken with Asparagus and Brown Rice*

Oven-baked chicken breast with roasted asparagus and a serving of brown rice.

Day 5

Breakfast
- *Cottage Cheese with Cherry Tomatoes and Cucumbers*

A bowl of low-fat cottage cheese with sliced cherry tomatoes and cucumber on the side.

Lunch
- *Tuna Salad with Mixed Greens*

Canned tuna mixed with olive oil, lemon juice, and mustard, served over mixed greens.

Dinner
- *Grilled Steak with Sautéed Spinach and Sweet Potato*

A lean cut of steak grilled and served with sautéed spinach and a small portion of roasted sweet potato.

Day 6

Breakfast
- *Protein powder, spinach, and almond milk in a smoothie*

a protein powder scoop, spinach, and almond milk combined to make a smoothie. Add a few frozen berries for sweetness.

Lunch
- *Quinoa Salad with Grilled Shrimp*

Quinoa mixed with grilled shrimp, cherry tomatoes, cucumber, and olive oil vinaigrette.

Dinner
- **Roasted Brussels Sprouts, Quinoa, and Baked Cod**

Cod fillets baked with herbs, served with roasted Brussels sprouts and cooked quinoa.

Day 7

Breakfast
Avocado Toast with Poached Eggs
Whole grain toast topped with mashed avocado and a poached egg, sprinkled with salt and pepper.

Lunch
- **Chicken Caesar Salad**

Grilled chicken breast served over romaine lettuce with a light Caesar dressing and a sprinkle of parmesan cheese.

Dinner
- **Grilled Salmon with Asparagus and Brown Rice**

A grilled salmon fillet paired with roasted asparagus and brown rice.

Day 8

Breakfast
- **Scrambled Eggs with Mushrooms and Onions**

Scrambled eggs with sautéed mushrooms and onions, served with a slice of whole grain toast.

Lunch
- **Avocado and Turkey Lettuce Wraps**

Sliced turkey and avocado wrapped in large lettuce leaves, with a drizzle of mustard or olive oil.

Dinner
- *Grilled Chicken with Steamed Broccoli and Cauliflower*

Grilled chicken served with a side of steamed broccoli and cauliflower.

Day 9

Breakfast
- *Greek Yogurt with Almond Butter and Chia Seeds*

A bowl of Greek yogurt mixed with almond butter and topped with chia seeds.

Lunch
- *Tuna Salad Lettuce Wraps*

Tuna salad (made with olive oil, lemon, and mustard) wrapped in large lettuce leaves.

Dinner
- *Baked Chicken with Quinoa and Roasted Vegetables*

Baked chicken breast served with quinoa and roasted mixed vegetables, including zucchini and bell peppers.

Day 10

Breakfast
- *Veggie Omelet with a Side of Avocado*

A veggie omelet made with bell peppers, onions, and spinach, served with half an avocado on the side.

Lunch
- Grilled Shrimp Salad with Lemon Vinaigrette

Grilled shrimp on a bed of mixed greens, with cucumbers, tomatoes, and a lemon vinaigrette dressing.

Dinner
- **Zucchini Noodles with Grilled Chicken and Tomato Sauce**

Zucchini noodles sautéed with olive oil and garlic, topped with homemade tomato sauce and grilled chicken.

Day 11

Breakfast
- **Cottage Cheese with Pineapple**

Low-fat cottage cheese topped with fresh pineapple chunks.

Lunch
- **Chicken and Veggie Stir-Fry**

Stir-fried chicken with mixed vegetables like bell peppers, broccoli, and onions, cooked in olive oil.

Dinner
- **Quinoa and Steamed Green Beans with Baked Salmon**

Baked salmon fillet served with steamed green beans and cooked quinoa.

Day 12

Breakfast
- **Chia Seed Pudding with Blueberries**

Almond milk-based chia seed pudding with fresh blueberries on top.

Lunch
- *Grilled Chicken with Avocado and Tomato Salad*

Grilled chicken breast served with a side of fresh tomato, avocado, and cucumber salad.

Dinner
- *Grilled Steak with Asparagus and Sweet Potato*

A lean steak grilled and paired with roasted asparagus and a small portion of sweet potato.

Day 13

Breakfast
- *Greek Yogurt with Walnuts and Honey*

Honey drizzled over plain Greek yogurt with chopped walnuts on top.

Lunch
- *Shrimp and Cucumber Salad*

Grilled shrimp served over a bed of cucumber and tomato salad, dressed with olive oil and lemon.

Dinner
- *Roasted cauliflower and Brussels sprouts with grilled chicken*

Roasted cauliflower and Brussels sprouts, seasoned with garlic and olive oil, accompany the grilled chicken.

Day 14

Breakfast
- *Scrambled Eggs with Bell Peppers and Onions*

Scrambled eggs with sautéed bell peppers and onions.

Lunch
- **Tuna Salad with Mixed Greens**

Canned tuna mixed with olive oil, mustard, and lemon juice, served over mixed greens.

Dinner
- **Baked Cod with Steamed Broccoli and Quinoa**

Cod fillets baked with herbs, served with steamed broccoli and cooked quinoa.

The Phase 2 recipes and meal plan in this chapter help maintain steady weight loss without sacrificing flavor or satisfaction. These meals are balanced with lean proteins, healthy fats, and plenty of vegetables, ensuring you stay full and energized. Enjoy the variety and flexibility these recipes provide as you continue your journey on the South Beach Diet.

CHAPTER 7
Phase 3 Recipes (Maintenance)

Phase 3 of the South Beach Diet is about maintaining your weight loss and establishing a healthy, sustainable way of eating. During this phase, you can reintroduce a wider variety of whole grains, legumes, and fruits into your meals while focusing on balanced and nutritious ingredients. Below are some delicious breakfast recipes that are not only easy to make but also support your maintenance goals with wholesome ingredients.

Sourdough French Toast with Fresh Fruit Compote
COOKING TIME: 15 MINUTES

SERVINGS: 2

Ingredients:
- 2 slices of whole grain sourdough bread
- 2 eggs
- 1/4 cup unsweetened almond milk
- 1/2 tsp vanilla extract
- 1/4 tsp ground cinnamon
- 1 tbsp olive oil or butter for cooking
- Fresh fruit for compote (strawberries, blueberries, and raspberries)
- 1 tbsp honey
- 1 tbsp lemon juice

Instructions:
- Put the lemon juice, honey, and mixed berries in a compact saucepan. Stirring occasionally, cook over low heat for five to seven minutes, or until the berries have released their juices and the mixture has somewhat thickened. Remove from heat.
- In a shallow dish, whisk together the eggs, almond milk, vanilla extract, and cinnamon.
- In a saucepan, melt the butter or olive oil over a moderate flame. Make sure to thoroughly coat each piece of sourdough bread by dipping it into the egg mixture. Cook each slice in the skillet for 2-3 minutes on each side, or until golden brown.
- Place the cooked French toast on plates and top with the fresh fruit compote. Serve immediately.

Whole Grain Breakfast Burrito with Sweet Potato Hash

COOKING TIME: 20 MINUTES

SERVINGS: 2

Ingredients:
- 2 whole grain tortillas
- 2 eggs
- 1/2 cup cooked sweet potato (diced)
- 1/4 cup red bell pepper (diced)
- 1/4 cup onion (diced)
- 1 tbsp olive oil
- 1/4 tsp chili powder
- Salt and pepper to taste
- 1/4 cup shredded cheese (optional)
- Fresh cilantro (for garnish)

Instructions:
- In a saucepan over a moderate flame, heat the olive oil. Add the bell pepper, onions, and sweet potato chopped. Stirring occasionally, cook the vegetables for five to seven minutes, or until they are tender and have a light brown. Now you can add some chili powder, salt, and pepper, and mix well.
- The eggs should be scrambled over medium heat in a different pan until they are done to your preference.
- Place a whole grain tortilla on each plate. Layer the sweet potato hash, scrambled eggs, and optional cheese. Roll up the tortillas into burritos.
- Garnish with fresh cilantro and serve immediately.

Avocado and Poached Egg Power Grain Bowl

COOKING TIME: 15 MINUTES

SERVINGS: 2

Ingredients:
- 1/2 cup quinoa (cooked)
- 1/2 cup cooked farro
- 2 eggs
- 1 ripe avocado, sliced
- 1 tbsp olive oil
- 1 tbsp lemon juice
- Salt and pepper to taste
- Fresh herbs for garnish (optional)

Instructions:
- If the quinoa and farro aren't already cooked, prepare them according to the package instructions.
- In a small pot of simmering water, gently add the eggs. Poach for about 4 minutes for a soft yolk, or longer if you prefer your eggs more done. Remove carefully from the water.
- Place the cooked farro and quinoa in a bowl. Drizzle with olive oil and lemon juice. Season with salt and pepper to taste.
- Place a poached egg on top of the grain mixture, then arrange sliced avocado around the egg.
- Serve right away, garnished with fresh herbs if preferred.

Multigrain Waffle with Greek Yogurt and Honey
COOKING TIME: 10 MINUTES
SERVINGS: 2

Ingredients:
- 1 cup multigrain waffle mix (or homemade recipe)
- 1/2 cup Greek yogurt (plain, non-fat)
- 1 tbsp honey
- Fresh berries for topping

Instructions:
- Follow the instructions on your multigrain waffle mix to make the waffles. Typically, this involves mixing the dry ingredients with water or milk, then cooking in a waffle iron for 3-5 minutes.
- While the waffles cook, place Greek yogurt in a small bowl and drizzle with honey. Stir gently to combine.
- Put the waffles on a plate when they're cooked. Add fresh berries, honey, and Greek yogurt on top.

Mediterranean Breakfast Pizza on Whole Grain Base

COOKING TIME: 20 MINUTES

SERVINGS: 2

Ingredients:
- 2 whole grain pita breads
- 2 tbsp olive oil
- 1/4 cup tomato sauce
- 1/2 cup shredded mozzarella cheese
- 1/4 cup kalamata olives, sliced
- 1/4 cup red onion, thinly sliced
- 1/4 cup cherry tomatoes, halved
- Fresh basil leaves (for garnish)

Instructions:
- Preheat your oven to 400°F (200°C). Place the whole grain pita breads on a baking sheet and drizzle each with olive oil.
- Spread a thin layer of tomato sauce on each pita, then sprinkle with shredded mozzarella. Top with olives, onions, and cherry tomatoes.
- Place the pizzas in the oven and bake for 8-10 minutes, or until the cheese is melted and the edges of the pita are crispy.
- Garnish with fresh basil leaves and serve immediately.

Banana Oat Pancakes with Almond Butter

COOKING TIME: 15 MINUTES

SERVINGS: 2

Ingredients:
- 1 ripe banana, mashed
- 1/2 cup rolled oats
- 2 eggs
- 1/4 tsp cinnamon
- 1/2 tsp vanilla extract
- 1 tbsp almond butter
- 1 tbsp coconut oil (for cooking)

Instructions:
- In a bowl, combine the mashed banana, oats, eggs, cinnamon, and vanilla extract. Mix until smooth.
- In a saucepan, heat the coconut oil over a medium-low flame. Pour the pancake batter into the skillet to form small pancakes. Cook until golden brown, approximately two to three minutes per side.
- Top with almond butter and serve immediately.

Breakfast Grain Bowl with Mango and Coconut

COOKING TIME: 10 MINUTES

SERVINGS: 2

Ingredients:
- 1/2 cup cooked brown rice
- 1/2 cup cooked quinoa
- 1/2 cup mango, diced
- 1/4 cup unsweetened coconut flakes
- 1 tbsp chia seeds
- 1 tbsp honey
- 1 tbsp lime juice

Instructions:
- If the brown rice and quinoa aren't cooked yet, cook them according to package instructions.
- In a bowl, combine the cooked grains. Top with diced mango, coconut flakes, chia seeds, and a drizzle of honey and lime juice.
- Mix well and serve immediately.

Ancient Grain Porridge with Caramelized Fruits

COOKING TIME: 20 MINUTES

SERVINGS: 2

Ingredients:
- 1/2 cup cooked ancient grains (like spelt or farro)
- 1/4 cup almond milk
- 1 tbsp honey
- 1/2 apple, thinly sliced
- 1/2 pear, thinly sliced
- 1 tbsp butter (for caramelizing)
- 1/4 tsp cinnamon

Instructions:
- Put the cooked oats and almond milk in a compact saucepan. Warm the porridge over a moderate flame, stirring periodically.
- Melt the butter in a separate pan over a medium-low flame. Add the apple and pear slices, sprinkle with cinnamon, and cook for 5-7 minutes until the fruits soften and caramelize.
- Transfer the heated porridge into bowls, garnish with honey, and add caramelized fruits on top.
- Serve immediately.

Ricotta Toast with Figs and Pistachios
COOKING TIME: 10 MINUTES
SERVINGS: 2

Ingredients:
- 2 slices whole grain bread
- 1/4 cup ricotta cheese
- 2 figs, sliced
- 1 tbsp pistachios, chopped
- 1 tsp honey
- Fresh mint for garnish (optional)

Instructions:
- The whole grain bread pieces should be toasted until golden brown.
- Evenly distribute ricotta cheese over each bread slice. Add chopped and sliced figs on top, drizzle with honey, and sprinkle with fresh mint. Serve immediately.

Green Power Smoothie Bowl with Granola

COOKING TIME: 10 MINUTES

SERVINGS: 2

Ingredients:
- 1 cup spinach
- 1/2 cup almond milk
- 1/2 banana
- 1/2 cup frozen mango
- 1 tbsp chia seeds
- 1/4 cup granola (unsweetened)

Instructions:
- Blend spinach, almond milk, banana, and mango until smooth.
- Pour the smoothie into bowls and top with chia seeds and granola. Serve immediately.

These recipes are perfect for maintaining your weight loss while keeping meals delicious and satisfying. Each one supports a balanced, healthy lifestyle with the right combination of protein, healthy fats, and complex carbs. Enjoy!

Lunch Recipes

As you move into Phase 3 of the South Beach Diet, your focus should shift towards maintaining your weight while continuing to enjoy healthy, balanced meals. In this phase, you can reintroduce more whole grains, legumes, and fruits. These recipes are designed to be delicious, satisfying, and simple to prepare—perfect for keeping you on track while enjoying a variety of flavors.

Mediterranean Grain Bowl with Grilled Halloumi

COOKING TIME: 20 MINUTES

SERVINGS: 2

Ingredients:
- 1 cup cooked quinoa
- 1/2 cup cherry tomatoes, halved
- 1/4 cup cucumber, diced
- 1/4 cup red onion, thinly sliced
- 1/4 cup Kalamata olives, pitted and sliced
- 1 tbsp olive oil
- 200g Halloumi cheese, sliced
- 1 tbsp fresh lemon juice
- 1 tbsp olive oil for grilling
- Fresh parsley, chopped (for garnish)

Instructions:
- Put the cooked quinoa, red onion, cucumber, cherry tomatoes, and olives in a bowl. Set aside.

- In a non-stick saucepan heat the olive oil over a medium-low flame. Add Halloumi slices and grill for about 2-3 minutes per side, until golden brown.
- Top the quinoa mixture with the grilled Halloumi, drizzle with lemon Enjoy this fresh, Mediterranean-inspired lunch.

Sesame Soba Noodle Salad with Seared Tuna

- **COOKING TIME: 15 MINUTES**
- **SERVINGS: 2**

Ingredients:
- 1 cup soba noodles
- 1 tbsp sesame oil
- 1 tbsp soy sauce (low sodium)
- 1 tsp honey
- 1 tsp rice vinegar
- 1 tsp sesame seeds
- 2 tuna steaks
- Salt and pepper to taste
- 1/4 cup green onions, chopped
- 1 tbsp toasted sesame seeds for garnish

Instructions:
- Follow the directions on the package to prepare the soba noodles. Drain and set aside to cool.
- In a small bowl, whisk together sesame oil, soy sauce, honey, rice vinegar, and sesame seeds.

- Season the tuna steaks with salt and pepper. Heat a pan over medium-high heat and sear the tuna for about 2-3 minutes per side for rare, or longer for your desired doneness.
- Toss the cooled soba noodles with the dressing. Slice the seared tuna and arrange it on top of the noodles.
- Garnish with green onions and toasted sesame seeds. Serve immediately.

Quinoa Power Bowl with Roasted Vegetables

COOKING TIME: 30 MINUTES

SERVINGS: 2

Ingredients:
- 1 cup cooked quinoa
- 1 small sweet potato, diced
- 1 cup broccoli florets
- 1/2 red bell pepper, sliced
- 1 tbsp olive oil
- 1 tsp ground cumin
- 1/2 tsp paprika
- Salt and pepper to taste
- 1/4 cup feta cheese, crumbled
- 1 tbsp tahini dressing

Instructions:
- Preheat your oven to 400°F (200°C). Toss the sweet potato, broccoli, and red bell pepper with olive oil, cumin, paprika, salt, and pepper. Arrange them on a baking sheet and bake for about twenty to twenty-five

minutes, or until they are soft and beginning to crisp up.
- While the vegetables roast, prepare the quinoa according to the package's instructions.
- In a bowl, combine the roasted vegetables and cooked quinoa. Top with crumbled feta cheese and drizzle with tahini dressing.
- Enjoy this nutrient-packed, colorful power bowl.

Whole Grain Pita with Falafel and Hummus
COOKING TIME: 20 MINUTES
SERVINGS: 2

Ingredients:
- 2 whole grain pita breads
- 6-8 falafel balls (store-bought or homemade)
- 1/2 cup hummus
- 1/4 cup cucumber, diced
- 1/4 cup tomato, diced
- 1/4 cup red onion, thinly sliced
- Fresh parsley for garnish

Instructions:
- Follow the directions on the package to reheat store-bought falafel. If making homemade, cook them as per your recipe.
- Warm the whole grain pita breads in the oven or on a skillet for 2-3 minutes.
- Each pita should have a thick layer of hummus on it. Add the cooked falafel, then top with diced cucumber, tomato, red onion, and fresh parsley.
- Enjoy this delicious Mediterranean-inspired lunch.

Asian-Style Rice Bowl with Teriyaki Chicken

COOKING TIME: 25 MINUTES

SERVINGS: 2

Ingredients:
- 1 cup brown rice, cooked
- 2 chicken breasts
- 1/4 cup teriyaki sauce (low sodium)
- 1 tbsp sesame oil
- 1/2 cup shredded carrots
- 1/4 cup edamame beans (steamed)
- 1 tbsp chopped green onions
- 1 tsp sesame seeds

Instructions:
- In a pan, heat the sesame oil over a medium- high flame. Cook the chicken breasts for six to seven minutes on each side, or until they are cooked through. In the final two minutes of cooking, drizzle the chicken with the teriyaki sauce.
- While the chicken is cooking, cook the brown rice and steam the edamame beans. Shred the carrots.
- Place a serving of rice in each bowl. Place the rice on top of the sliced teriyaki chicken. Add shredded carrots and steamed edamame.
- Garnish with green onions and sesame seeds. Serve immediately.

Southwest Black Bean and Corn Salad

COOKING TIME: 15 MINUTES

SERVINGS: 2

Ingredients:
- 1 cup cooked black beans
- 1/2 cup corn kernels (fresh or frozen)
- 1/4 cup red bell pepper, diced
- 1/4 cup red onion, diced
- 1 tbsp olive oil
- 1 tbsp lime juice
- 1 tsp cumin
- Salt and pepper to taste
- Fresh cilantro, chopped

Instructions:
- In a bowl, combine black beans, corn, red bell pepper, and red onion.
- Mix the lime juice, cumin, olive oil, salt, and pepper in another bowl.
- After adding the dressing to the salad, toss to mix everything together.
- Garnish with fresh cilantro and serve immediately.

Grilled Vegetable and Couscous Bowl

COOKING TIME: 20 MINUTES

SERVINGS: 2

Ingredients:
- 1 cup cooked couscous
- 1 zucchini, sliced
- 1 eggplant, sliced
- 1 bell pepper, sliced
- 1 tbsp olive oil
- Salt and pepper to taste
- 1 tbsp balsamic vinegar
- Fresh basil, chopped (for garnish)

Instructions:
- Set the temperature of your grill or grill pan to medium-high temperature. Add salt, pepper, and olive oil to the bell pepper, zucchini, and eggplant. Grill until soft and gently charred, about five to seven minutes, flipping periodically.
- Cook the couscous according to the package instructions.
- Place the couscous in bowls and top with the grilled vegetables. Drizzle with balsamic vinegar.
- Garnish with fresh basil and serve immediately.

Turkey and Avocado California Wrap

COOKING TIME: 10 MINUTES

SERVINGS: 2

Ingredients:
- 2 whole wheat tortillas
- 4 slices turkey breast (lean)
- 1/2 avocado, sliced
- 1/4 cup spinach leaves
- 1 tbsp mustard or hummus (optional)
- Salt and pepper to taste

Instructions:
- Lay the tortillas flat. Place turkey slices, avocado, and spinach leaves in the center of each tortilla. Add mustard or hummus if desired.
- Sprinkle with salt and pepper, then roll up the tortillas tightly.
- Slice the wraps in half and serve immediately.

Mediterranean Tuna Nicoise with Potatoes

COOKING TIME: 30 MINUTES

SERVINGS: 2

Ingredients:
- 1 can tuna (in olive oil, drained)
- 4 small new potatoes, boiled and halved
- 1/2 cup green beans, steamed
- 1/4 cup black olives
- 1 boiled egg, quartered
- 1 tbsp olive oil
- 1 tbsp red wine vinegar
- 1 tsp Dijon mustard
- Salt and pepper to taste

Instructions:
- In a bowl, combine the tuna, boiled potatoes, steamed green beans, black olives, and boiled egg.
- Mix the olive oil, Dijon mustard, red wine vinegar, salt, and pepper in another bowl.
- Sprinkle the salad with the dressing and gently toss to mix.
- Enjoy this fresh Mediterranean salad immediately.

Chickpea and Sweet Potato Buddha Bowl

COOKING TIME: 30 MINUTES

SERVINGS: 2

Ingredients:
- 1 cup cooked chickpeas
- 1 small sweet potato, cubed
- 1 tbsp olive oil
- 1 tsp smoked paprika
- 1/2 avocado, sliced
- 1/4 cup cucumber, diced
- 1 tbsp tahini dressing

Instructions:
- Preheat the oven to 400°F (200°C). Toss the sweet potato cubes with olive oil and smoked paprika. Roast for 20-25 minutes until tender and crispy.
- In a bowl, combine cooked chickpeas, roasted sweet potatoes, avocado, and cucumber.
- Drizzle with tahini dressing and serve immediately.

These lunch recipes for Phase 3 are not only easy to make but also full of flavor and nutrients that will help you maintain your weight while enjoying every bite.

Dinner Recipes

Maintaining a healthy weight doesn't mean you need to sacrifice flavor or variety in your meals. These dinner recipes are designed to help you stay satisfied while supporting your goal of weight maintenance. Enjoy these simple yet delicious dishes that are packed with nutrients and offer a perfect balance of protein, fiber, and healthy fats.

Honey-Glazed Salmon with Wild Rice Pilaf
COOKING TIME: 30 MINUTES
SERVINGS: 2

Ingredients:
- 2 salmon fillets
- 1 tbsp honey
- 1 tbsp Dijon mustard
- 1 tbsp olive oil
- 1/2 cup wild rice
- 1 cup vegetable broth
- 1/4 cup diced red onion
- 1/4 cup chopped parsley
- Salt and pepper to taste

Instructions:
- Preheat the oven to 375°F (190°C). Combine honey, olive oil, Dijon mustard, salt, and pepper in a small bowl.
- Place the salmon fillets on a baking sheet. Drizzle the fillets with the honey-mustard glaze.

- The salmon should be cooked through and flake readily with a fork after about fifteen to twenty minutes in the oven.
- While the salmon is baking, bring vegetable broth to a boil in a medium saucepan. Add the wild rice, reduce heat, and simmer for 20-25 minutes, until the rice is tender and the broth is absorbed.
- In a separate pan, sauté the diced red onion in a little olive oil until soft. Add chopped parsley and cooked rice, and stir. Season with salt and pepper.
- Serve the glazed salmon over the wild rice pilaf and enjoy!

Mediterranean Chicken with Pearl Couscous

COOKING TIME: 35 MINUTES
SERVINGS: 2

Ingredients:
- 2 boneless, skinless chicken breasts
- 1 tbsp olive oil
- 1 tsp dried oregano
- 1/2 tsp garlic powder
- 1/4 tsp salt
- 1/4 tsp black pepper
- 1/2 cup pearl couscous
- 1 cup vegetable broth
- 1/2 cup cherry tomatoes, halved
- 1/4 cup Kalamata olives, chopped
- 1/4 cup crumbled feta cheese

Instructions:
- Add salt, pepper, garlic powder, oregano, and olive oil to the chicken breasts.
- A saucepan or grill pan should be heated to moderate temperature. Bring the internal temperature of the chicken to 165°F (74°C) after cooking it for between 6 and 7 minutes on each side.
- While the chicken cooks, bring vegetable broth to a boil in a saucepan. Add the pearl couscous, reduce heat, and simmer for 10 minutes until tender and the broth is absorbed.
- Once the couscous is cooked, stir in the cherry tomatoes, olives, and feta cheese.
- Slice the chicken and serve over the couscous mixture.

Grass-Fed Beef Stir-Fry with Brown Rice
COOKING TIME: 25 MINUTES
SERVINGS: 2

Ingredients:
- 1/2 lb grass-fed beef, thinly sliced
- 1 tbsp sesame oil
- 1/2 cup sliced bell peppers (red, yellow, green)
- 1/2 cup sliced onions
- 1/2 cup snap peas
- 2 tbsp soy sauce (or tamari for gluten-free)
- 1 tbsp rice vinegar
- 1 tsp honey
- 1 cup cooked brown rice
- 1 tbsp sesame seeds

Instructions:
- Mix the rice vinegar, honey, and soy sauce in a small basin.
- In an extensive pan or wok, heat the sesame oil over a medium- high flame. Cook the beef slices for about three to four minutes, stirring often, until they are browned.
- Add the bell peppers, onions, and snap peas to the pan. The vegetables should be crisp-tender after another three to four minutes of stirring.
- Cover the steak and veggies with the stir-fry sauce. Stir to coat evenly. Cook for another minute.
- Serve the beef stir-fry over a bed of brown rice and sprinkle with sesame seeds.

Baked Fish with Ancient Grain Risotto

COOKING TIME: 40 MINUTES
SERVINGS: 2

Ingredients:

- Two fillets of white fish, such haddock or cod
- 1 tbsp olive oil
- 1 tsp lemon zest
- 1 tbsp fresh lemon juice
- Salt and pepper to taste
- 1/2 cup ancient grains (quinoa, farro, or spelt)
- 1 cup vegetable broth
- 1/4 cup grated Parmesan cheese
- 1/4 cup chopped parsley

Instructions:

- Preheat the oven to 375°F (190°C). Place the fish fillets on a baking sheet and drizzle with olive oil, lemon zest, and lemon juice. Season with salt and pepper. Bake until the fish flakes easily, about fifteen to twenty minutes.
- Heat the veggie broth in a saucepan until it boils. Add the ancient grains and reduce the heat. Simmer for 15-20 minutes, or until tender and the broth is absorbed.
- Stir in the Parmesan cheese and chopped parsley into the cooked grains.
- Plate the baked fish and serve alongside the ancient grain risotto.

Turkey and Quinoa Stuffed Acorn Squash

COOKING TIME: 45 MINUTES

SERVINGS: 2

Ingredients:
- 2 acorn squashes, halved and seeds removed
- 1 tbsp olive oil
- 1/2 lb ground turkey
- 1/2 cup cooked quinoa
- 1/4 cup chopped onions
- 1/4 cup chopped spinach
- 1/4 cup crumbled feta cheese
- Salt and pepper to taste

Instructions:
- Preheat the oven to 375°F (190°C). Season the acorn squash with salt and pepper after drizzling it with olive oil on the sliced sides. Place the squash cut side down on a baking sheet and bake for thirty-thirty-five minutes, or until tender.
- In a skillet over medium heat, cook the ground turkey with the onions until browned and cooked through.
- Stir in the cooked quinoa and chopped spinach to the turkey mixture. Season with salt and pepper.
- Once the acorn squash is cooked, stuff each half with the turkey-quinoa mixture. Top with crumbled feta cheese.
- Serve the stuffed squash warm.

Shrimp and Whole Grain Pasta with Pesto

COOKING TIME: 20 MINUTES

SERVINGS: 2

Ingredients:
- 1/2 lb shrimp, peeled and deveined
- 4 oz whole grain pasta
- 1/4 cup pesto sauce
- 1 tbsp olive oil
- 1/4 cup cherry tomatoes, halved
- Salt and pepper to taste

Instructions:
- Follow the directions on the package to prepare the whole grain pasta. Drain and set aside.
- Olive oil should be heated in a saucepan over a moderate temperature. Add the shrimp and fry until cooked through and pink, two to three minutes per side.
- Add the cooked pasta and pesto sauce to the skillet with the shrimp. Toss to combine.
- Top with halved cherry tomatoes and serve immediately.

Lamb Chops with Mediterranean Grain Salad
COOKING TIME: 40 MINUTES
SERVINGS: 2

Ingredients:
- 2 lamb chops
- 1 tbsp olive oil
- 1 tsp rosemary
- 1/2 cup cooked farro
- 1/4 cup diced cucumber
- 1/4 cup cherry tomatoes, halved
- 1/4 cup Kalamata olives, chopped
- 1/4 cup crumbled feta cheese

Instructions:
- Preheat the grill or skillet over medium-high heat. Rub the lamb chops with olive oil and rosemary. For medium-rare, grill for about four to five minutes on each side; if you want it more done, grill for longer.
- In a bowl, combine cooked farro, cucumber, tomatoes, olives, and feta cheese. Toss to combine.
- Serve the lamb chops alongside the Mediterranean grain salad.

Asian-Inspired Rice Bowl with Tofu

COOKING TIME: 25 MINUTES

SERVINGS: 2

Ingredients:

- 1/2 lb firm tofu, cubed
- 1 tbsp sesame oil
- 1/2 cup cooked brown rice
- 1/4 cup shredded carrots
- 1/4 cup sliced cucumber
- 2 tbsp soy sauce
- 1 tsp rice vinegar
- 1/4 tsp sesame seeds

Instructions:

- In a pan, heat the sesame oil over a moderate flame. Add tofu cubes and cook for 5-7 minutes until crispy and golden.
- In a bowl, layer the cooked brown rice, shredded carrots, sliced cucumber, and cooked tofu.
- Drizzle with soy sauce and rice vinegar, and top with sesame seeds.

Grilled Chicken with Sweet Potato Mash

COOKING TIME: 30 MINUTES

SERVINGS: 2

Ingredients:
- 2 boneless, skinless chicken breasts
- 1 tbsp olive oil
- 1/2 tsp paprika
- 1/2 tsp garlic powder
- 1 large sweet potato, peeled and cubed
- 1 tbsp butter
- Salt and pepper to taste

Instructions:
- Add salt, pepper, garlic powder, paprika, and olive oil to the chicken breasts. Grill over medium heat for 6-7 minutes per side.
- Boil the cubed sweet potato in salted water for 10-12 minutes until tender. After draining, mash with salt, pepper, and butter.
- Serve sweet potato mash beside the grilled chicken.

Seafood Paella with Brown Rice

COOKING TIME: 40 MINUTES

SERVINGS: 2

Ingredients:

- 1/2 lb mixed seafood (shrimp, mussels, squid)
- 1 tbsp olive oil
- 1/2 cup chopped onion
- 1/2 cup bell peppers, chopped
- 1/2 tsp smoked paprika
- 1/2 cup cooked brown rice
- 1/4 cup peas
- 1 tbsp fresh parsley

Instructions:

- In a large pan, heat the olive oil over a moderate flame. Add the seafood and cook until opaque and cooked through, about 4-5 minutes.
- Add the bell peppers and onion to the same pan and cook for approximately three to four minutes. Stir in smoked paprika.
- Add the cooked brown rice and peas. Stir well and cook for 5 minutes.
- Top with fresh parsley and serve.

These dinner recipes are designed to keep your meals fresh, exciting, and aligned with the South Beach Diet Phase 3 principles. Whether you're in the mood for seafood, chicken, or plant-based options, there's something here to suit every taste.

Approved Snacks

Here are 15 approved snacks to enjoy during Phase 3 of the South Beach Diet. These snacks are nutrient-dense, delicious, and balanced, supporting your weight management goals while keeping you satisfied:

- Greek yogurt with chia seeds and honey
- Sliced apple with almond butter
- Roasted chickpeas
- Carrot sticks with hummus
- Celery sticks with peanut butter
- Hard-boiled eggs with a pinch of sea salt
- Sliced cucumber with guacamole
- Cottage cheese with sliced peaches
- Almonds and a handful of dried cranberries
- Mixed berries with whipped coconut cream
- Rice cakes with avocado and tomato
- Edamame with a sprinkle of sea salt
- Roasted sunflower seeds
- Bell pepper strips with tzatziki
- Homemade granola bars

Meal Plans (14-Day Plan)

Below is a 14-day meal plan for Phase 3, with breakfast, lunch, and dinner options. This plan includes a variety of whole grains, lean proteins, healthy fats, and fresh vegetables, all while maintaining the balance that the South Beach Diet encourages.

Day 1
Breakfast: Whole Grain Breakfast Burrito with Sweet Potato Hash
Lunch: Mediterranean Grain Bowl with Grilled Halloumi
Dinner: Honey-Glazed Salmon with Wild Rice Pilaf

Day 2
Breakfast: Power Grain Bowl with Poached Egg and Avocado
Lunch: Quinoa Power Bowl with Roasted Vegetables
Dinner: Mediterranean Chicken with Pearl Couscous

Day 3
Breakfast: Multigrain Waffle with Greek Yogurt and Honey
Lunch: Sesame Soba Noodle Salad with Seared Tuna
Dinner: Grass-Fed Beef Stir-Fry with Brown Rice

Day 4
Breakfast: Banana Oat Pancakes with Almond Butter
Lunch: Whole Grain Pita with Falafel and Hummus
Dinner: Baked Fish with Ancient Grain Risotto

Day 5
Breakfast: Breakfast Grain Bowl with Mango and Coconut
Lunch: Asian-Style Rice Bowl with Teriyaki Chicken
Dinner: Turkey and Quinoa Stuffed Acorn Squash

Day 6
Breakfast: Ancient Grain Porridge with Caramelized Fruits
Lunch: Southwest Black Bean and Corn Salad
Dinner: Shrimp and Whole Grain Pasta with Pesto

Day 7
Breakfast: Ricotta Toast with Figs and Pistachios
Lunch: Grilled Vegetable and Couscous Bowl
Dinner: Lamb Chops with Mediterranean Grain Salad

Day 8
Breakfast: Green Power Smoothie Bowl with Granola
Lunch: Turkey and Avocado California Wrap
Dinner: Asian-Inspired Rice Bowl with Tofu

Day 9
Breakfast: Sourdough French Toast with Fresh Fruit Compote
Lunch: Mediterranean Tuna Niçoise with Potatoes
Dinner: Grilled Chicken with Sweet Potato Mash

Day 10
Breakfast: Whole Grain Breakfast Burrito with Sweet Potato Hash
Lunch: Chickpea and Sweet Potato Buddha Bowl
Dinner: Seafood Paella with Brown Rice

Day 11
Breakfast: Power Grain Bowl with Poached Egg and Avocado
Lunch: Quinoa Power Bowl with Roasted Vegetables
Dinner: Honey-Glazed Salmon with Wild Rice Pilaf

Day 12
Breakfast: Multigrain Waffle with Greek Yogurt and Honey
Lunch: Sesame Soba Noodle Salad with Seared Tuna
Dinner: Mediterranean Chicken with Pearl Couscous

Day 13
Breakfast: Banana Oat Pancakes with Almond Butter
Lunch: Whole Grain Pita with Falafel and Hummus
Dinner: Grass-Fed Beef Stir-Fry with Brown Rice

Day 14
Breakfast: Breakfast Grain Bowl with Mango and Coconut
Lunch: Southwest Black Bean and Corn Salad
Dinner: Turkey and Quinoa Stuffed Acorn Squash

These are just a few of the delicious and satisfying meals you can enjoy in Phase 3 of the South Beach Diet. This meal plan, combined with a variety of approved snacks, will help you maintain your weight loss and keep your body energized and nourished.

PART THREE: MASTERING THE LIFESTYLE

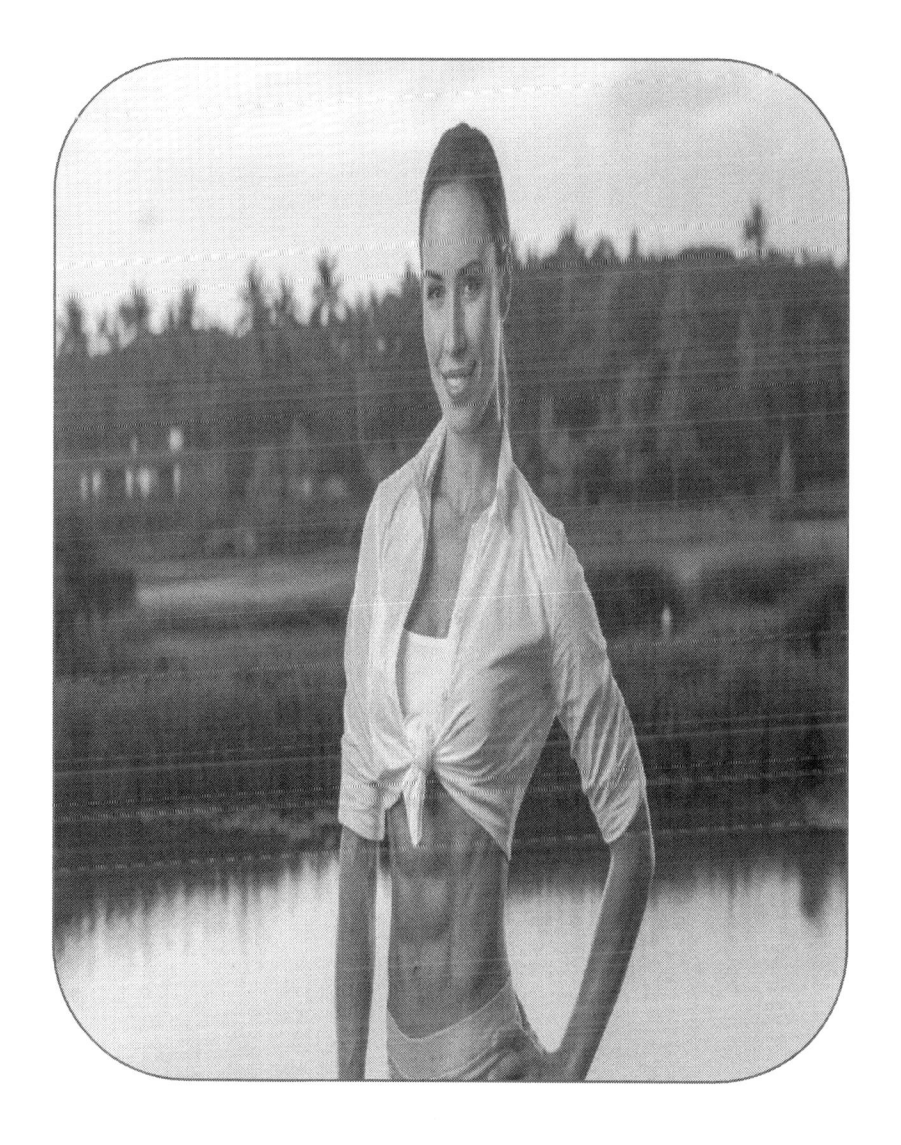

CHAPTER 8
Common Myths and Facts

When it comes to weight loss, the South Beach Diet has helped countless individuals achieve their goals through simple, healthy eating. However, along the way, many myths about diets and weight loss persist. In this chapter, we will debunk some of the most common myths, provide facts, and share real success stories to help you stay motivated and focused. Let's also dive into some troubleshooting tips to help you overcome obstacles.

Debunking Popular Diet Myths

Myth 1: Carbs are Bad for You

One of the most persistent myths in the world of dieting is that carbs are bad and should be avoided completely. This couldn't be further from the truth, especially on the South Beach Diet. The South Beach Diet focuses on good carbs — whole grains, fruits, and vegetables — while minimizing bad carbs from processed foods and sugars.

The key difference is the type of carbs you consume. Good carbs are nutrient-dense and help maintain steady blood sugar levels, which is important for energy and weight management. By choosing healthy carbs and balancing them with protein and healthy fats, you're not only fueling your body correctly but also avoiding the blood sugar spikes and crashes that contribute to weight gain.

Myth 2: You Have to Exercise Excessively to Lose Weight

Exercise is undoubtedly important for overall health, but you don't have to kill yourself in the gym to lose weight. Moderate physical activity and a balanced diet are key components of the South Beach Diet. You can see results without hours of intense exercise.

Regular physical activity, such as walking, swimming, or a moderate gym routine, combined with healthy eating habits, will yield results. You don't need extreme workout regimens to burn fat; a healthy, sustainable lifestyle is key.

Myth 3: Fats Make You Fat

This myth has been around for decades, but it's time to put it to rest. Not all fats are created equal. The South Beach Diet promotes the consumption of healthy fats, such as those found in avocado, nuts, olive oil, and fatty fish like salmon. These fats are essential for good health, supporting everything from brain function to hormone regulation.

Trans fats and saturated fats found in processed foods, however, should be avoided, as they can contribute to weight gain and increase your risk of heart disease. So, it's not about fat being inherently bad, but about making the right choices.

Myth 4: Calorie counting is necessary for weight loss.

Calorie counting can be helpful for some people, but it's not a necessity for success on the South Beach Diet. The key to weight loss is eating balanced meals with the right portions, not obsessing over each calorie. By focusing on whole, nutrient-dense foods that keep you satisfied, you can avoid overeating without having to count every calorie.

The South Beach Diet's meal planning system encourages eating whole foods and pairing them with protein and healthy fats to reduce hunger and prevent cravings. This approach makes it easier to maintain a healthy weight without calorie obsession.

Myth 5: You Can't Eat Your Favorite Foods While Dieting

This myth is one of the biggest reasons people struggle with diets. People often think they have to give up their favorite foods in order to lose weight, but that's not true. On the South Beach Diet, you can still enjoy foods like pasta, bread, and even desserts — but they need to be the right kind of foods.

The key is moderation and making healthier choices. For example, instead of white pasta, opt for whole grain or gluten-free pasta. Enjoy your favorite foods by swapping out ingredients to make them healthier while still satisfying your cravings. It's all about finding balance, not restriction.

Myth 6: You Can't Lose Weight Without Cutting Out All Sugar

While it's true that cutting down on sugar is important for weight loss, you don't need to eliminate all sugar from your life. The South Beach Diet encourages you to reduce the consumption of added sugars and highly processed sweet foods, which can spike insulin and lead to weight gain.

However, natural sugars found in fruits, vegetables, and whole grains are perfectly fine in moderation. These natural sugars come with fiber and other nutrients that make them a healthy part of your diet. You can still satisfy your sweet tooth with things like fruit-based desserts, dark chocolate, and other low-sugar options.

Success Stories

Real-life success stories are a powerful motivator for anyone starting or continuing the South Beach Diet. Here are just a few examples of people who have transformed their health and lives by following the principles of the South Beach Diet.

Emily's Transformation: From Stuck to Energized

For years, Emily, a 35-year-old mother of two, battled her weight. She made the decision to pursue the South Beach Diet after attempting several diets without seeing any permanent effects. "This diet's balance is what I love about it," she explains. I never felt deprived and was able to savor delectable meals. The meals were simple to prepare, and the meal plans were straightforward to follow.

Within just three months, Emily lost 25 pounds and noticed a huge improvement in her energy levels. She claims, "I feel like a new person." "My vitality is what truly leaps out, but the weight loss was the apparent advantage. I can now keep up with my children, and I no longer feel lethargic by noon.

Mark's Journey: Shedding 50 Pounds and Finding Confidence

Mark, a 42-year-old office worker, had struggled with obesity for most of his adult life. He decided to make a change after seeing a doctor who expressed concern about his rising cholesterol levels. After starting the South Beach Diet, Mark lost 50 pounds in just six months.

"The flexibility of the South Beach Diet was key for me," Mark says. "I didn't have to give up all the foods I loved, but I learned how to eat them in a healthier way. The combination of eating the right foods and losing weight helped me get off my cholesterol medication and feel better overall."

Mark also become more self-assured. "In both my personal and professional lives, I believe I have more space to develop. For me, losing weight was not as crucial as regaining my health.

Sophia's Success: Overcoming Plateaus
Sophia, 29, hit a weight-loss plateau after losing 25 pounds on the South Beach Diet. Feeling discouraged, she considered giving up. However, she decided to reach out for guidance and discovered that changing up her exercise routine and adjusting her meals helped her break through the plateau. "Believe me when I say, There are times when you just need to make a couple of minor adjustments," she explains. "The weight began to drop again after I changed up my workouts and increased the variety of my meals."

Sophia ultimately lost a total of 40 pounds and maintained her weight for over a year. "Trust me, I've really learned a lot about how to recharge my body in the right way. Now I solely focus on consistency, not just perfection."

Troubleshooting Guide

While following the South Beach Diet, you may encounter challenges that make weight loss feel difficult. Here are some common issues and practical tips for troubleshooting:

- *Problem 1: Stagnant Weight Loss*

It's common for weight loss to slow down or plateau after a period of success. If this happens, try the following:

Adjust Your Carb Intake: If you've been on Phase 2 for a while, you might need to reduce your carb intake slightly to get things moving again. Consider cutting out some starchy vegetables and reducing your whole grain portions.

Increase Your Physical Activity: If you've been doing light exercise, consider increasing the intensity or incorporating new activities like strength training or interval workouts.

Check for Hidden Sugar: Even small amounts of sugar from sauces, dressings, and snacks can add up. Reevaluate what you're eating to make sure hidden sugars aren't stalling your progress.

- *Problem 2: Cravings and Hunger*

If you're feeling hungry between meals or experiencing cravings, consider these tips:

Add More Protein and Fiber: Fiber and protein both contribute to a longer feeling of fullness. Incorporate veggies, beans, eggs, and lean meats into your meals.

Drink More Water: Thirst can occasionally be confused with hunger. Drink a full glass of water before you decide on reaching for a snack to see if your cravings would subside.

Plan Your Snacks: Keep healthy snacks like nuts, seeds, or veggie sticks on hand so you're not tempted to grab unhealthy options.

- ***Problem 3: Feeling Deprived***

The South Beach Diet is all about balance, not deprivation. If you're feeling deprived, try these strategies:

Find Healthier Substitutes: Missing a favorite food? Try healthier swaps. Craving pizza? Opt for a cauliflower crust. Want something sweet? Reach for dark chocolate or homemade fruit-based desserts.

Mindful Eating: Don't be in a rush, take your time and enjoy your food. By doing this, you can avoid overindulging and feel more content.

By addressing these common obstacles and staying consistent, you can keep your weight loss on track and maintain your progress.

Debunking these myths and embracing the facts will help you feel more confident in your weight loss journey. The South Beach Diet provides a flexible, sustainable approach to healthy eating, and the real-life success stories prove that it works. By sticking with the plan, making adjustments when necessary, and using the troubleshooting guide, you'll overcome challenges and reach your goals.

CHAPTER 9
Frequently Asked Questions

As you journey through the South Beach Diet, it's normal to have questions. This chapter will address some of the most common ones about general diet concerns, recipe modifications, special dietary needs, and weight loss plateaus. Whether you're just starting or are a seasoned dieter, this section will help you navigate challenges and make your experience easier.

General Diet Questions

Q1: Can I eat out while on the South Beach Diet?

Yes! One of the great things about the South Beach Diet is that it doesn't require you to be stuck at home. Eating out can still fit into your diet, as long as you make smart choices. A few pointers for eating out are as follows:

- **Choose Lean Proteins**: Opt for grilled chicken, fish, or turkey. Avoid fried items or those with heavy sauces.
- **Watch the Carbs**: Stick to non-starchy vegetables, and ask for a side salad instead of mashed potatoes or fries.
- **Be Mindful of Dressings and Sauces:** These can be loaded with sugar and fat. Use them sparingly and request them on the side.
- **Drink Water or Unsweetened Beverages**: Avoid sugary drinks and cocktails. Stick with water, iced tea, or coffee without added sugar.

With a little effort in planning, eating out doesn't really have to sabotage your diet.

Q2: How can I stay on track during holidays or special events?
Special occasions and holidays might be difficult, but they don't have to stop you from moving on. Here's how to stay on track:

- **Plan Ahead:** If you know you'll be attending a party, eat a healthy snack beforehand to avoid overeating.
- **Portion Control:** Enjoy the foods you love, but keep your portions in check. Focus on protein and veggies and limit carb-heavy foods.
- **Practice Mindful Eating:** Eat slowly, take it gently and savor your food while in your mouth. This can help you feel satisfied with less.
- **Stay Active:** Take a walk after the event or find ways to stay active during the day to balance out any extra calories.

By preparing and practicing moderation, you can navigate any special occasion without feeling guilty.

Q3: Can I drink alcohol on the South Beach Diet?
Yes, you can drink alcohol, but in moderation and with some guidelines. During Phase 1, it's best to avoid alcohol, as it can interfere with your body's ability to burn fat. In Phase 2 and beyond, you can reintroduce alcohol. Here are some guidelines:

- **Limit Alcohol to One Drink:** Stick with low-carb options like a glass of dry wine or a clear spirit like vodka or gin mixed with soda water.

- **Avoid Sugary Cocktails:** Mixed drinks like margaritas or pina coladas are loaded with sugar and carbs, so it's best to skip them.
- **Drink Water:** Alternate alcoholic drinks with water to stay hydrated and avoid overindulgence.

It's okay to occasionally enjoy a drink, but moderation is essential.

Q4: How do I know if I'm in Phase 1 or Phase 2 of the South Beach Diet?
Phase 1 is the initial two-week phase of the South Beach Diet, where you'll eliminate most carbs to reset your body. During this phase, you'll focus on high-protein foods like lean meats, fish, and eggs, along with non-starchy vegetables. No bread, pasta, or fruit are allowed.

Phase 2 introduces healthy, whole grains, fruit, and more variety to your meals. You'll gradually reintroduce certain carbs like berries, legumes, and whole grains, all while continuing to eat lean proteins and healthy fats. This phase lasts until you've reached your goal weight, and then you'll transition to Phase 3, which focuses on maintaining your weight.

Recipe Modifications

Q1: Can I modify the recipes to suit my taste or dietary preferences?
Absolutely! The South Beach Diet encourages flexibility, and recipes can be easily modified to suit your preferences. Here are some common modifications:

- *Swap Proteins:* If you don't like chicken, try turkey, lean beef, or tofu as a protein source.
- *Modify Vegetables:* Not a fan of spinach? No worries, you can use kale, arugula, or another leafy green instead. The South Beach Diet encourages a wide variety of vegetables, so feel free to experiment.
- *Adjust Seasonings:* If you prefer spicier food, add more herbs and spices. Fresh garlic, ginger, chili flakes, or lemon zest can add flavor without extra calories.
- *Healthy Swaps:* If a recipe calls for cheese, you can substitute with lower-fat cheese or skip it entirely. Similarly, use whole grain alternatives for any carb-heavy ingredients.

The beauty of the South Beach Diet is that it's adaptable to your tastes and preferences. Don't hesitate to modify recipes to make them your own.

Q2: Can I make these recipes for my family or guests?
Yes! Most South Beach Diet recipes are family-friendly and can be scaled up to serve more people. The meals are balanced and nutritious, making them a great option for anyone in the family, not just those following the diet. Here are a few tips for cooking for a group:

- *Prepare in Bulk:* Many South Beach Diet recipes, like soups, stews, and casseroles, can be made in larger quantities. You can also meal prep for the week as this will help you to save time.

- *Offer Variety:* While you may be focused on the South Beach guidelines, you can still offer guests a variety of dishes. For example, serve a healthy salad alongside a more traditional dish for those not following the diet.
- *Keep Things Simple:* Don't overcomplicate the meal. A few simple, healthy dishes will be more than enough.

The South Beach Diet doesn't require you to make separate meals for yourself. Most recipes can be adapted to feed everyone.

Q3: Can I make desserts on the South Beach Diet?

Oh Yes! You don't have to give up your sweet cravings on the South Beach Diet. Phase 1 limits desserts, but as you move into Phase 2 and 3, you can enjoy healthier versions of desserts. Here are some ideas:

- *Fruit-Based Desserts:* Fresh berries with a bit of whipped cream or Greek yogurt make a delicious and healthy dessert.
- *Dark Chocolate:* A small square of high-quality dark chocolate is allowed in moderation.
- *Homemade Treats:* Look for recipes that use almond flour, coconut flour, or stevia to make low-carb baked goods.

Desserts don't have to be full of sugar and empty calories. Choosing healthier options and exercising moderation are crucial.

Special Dietary Needs

Q1: Can I follow the South Beach Diet if I'm vegetarian or vegan?

Yes, the South Beach Diet can be easily modified for vegetarian or vegan lifestyles. Here are a few tips:

- *Focus on Plant-Based Proteins:* For vegetarians, beans, lentils, tofu, tempeh, and seitan are great protein sources. For vegans, tofu and tempeh are particularly useful.
- *Incorporate More Healthy Fats:* Avocados, nuts, seeds, and olive oil are all amazing great sources of healthy fats.
- *Choose Whole Grains:* Quinoa, brown rice, and oats are great carb options that fit within the South Beach Diet's guidelines.

The South Beach Diet is flexible enough to accommodate plant-based diets without sacrificing the principles of healthy eating.

Q2: Can I follow the South Beach Diet if I have food allergies?

Yes, the South Beach Diet can be adapted for people with various food allergies. Here's how you can adjust:

- *Dairy-Free:* If you're lactose intolerant, look for dairy alternatives like almond milk, coconut milk, or soy milk. Many recipes can be modified to be dairy-free without compromising flavor.
- *Gluten-Free:* For those who need to avoid gluten, there are plenty of gluten-free alternatives available, such as

gluten-free bread, pasta, and flour. Many South Beach Diet recipes already use gluten-free ingredients.
- *Nut-Free:* If you have a nut allergy, replace nut-based products with seeds (like chia, flax, or sunflower seeds) or non-nut butters like sunflower seed butter.

The South Beach Diet is all about choosing healthy ingredients that work for your body. You can easily adjust the recipes to fit your specific needs.

Weight Loss Plateaus

Q1: What should I do if I hit a weight loss plateau?
Anyone can experience weight reduction plateaus, which are a common occurrence during the process. Here are some techniques to assist you get past a plateau if you're stuck:

- *Reevaluate Your Portions:* Even healthy foods can contribute to weight gain if you eat them in large quantities. Make sure you're following the portion sizes recommended for the South Beach Diet.
- *Increase Your Physical Activity:* Adding strength training or high-intensity interval training (HIIT) can help rev up your metabolism and break through a plateau.
- *Reduce Carbs Temporarily:* If you've reached Phase 2 or 3, cutting back on your carb intake for a short period can help your body reset and jump-start weight loss again.

- ***Ensure Adequate Sleep:*** Poor sleep can contribute to weight loss plateaus, so make sure you're getting 7-9 hours of sleep each night.

Plateaus are frustrating, but with patience and consistency, you can overcome them and continue making progress toward your weight loss goals.

Q2: How long should I stay in each phase?
Phase 1 lasts for two weeks, and during this time, your body will go through a reset. After Phase 1, you can move on to Phase 2, where you'll begin to reintroduce some healthy carbs like whole grains and fruits. You'll stay in Phase 2 until you've reached your target weight. Finally, Phase 3 is your maintenance phase, where you'll focus on keeping the weight off and maintaining a healthy, balanced lifestyle.

It's important to listen to your body. If you're feeling good and progressing well, there's no need to rush through the phases. Take your time to adjust as needed.

CONCLUSION
Your Lifelong Journey

Losing weight is only one aspect of adopting a healthy lifestyle with the South Beach Diet; another is embracing a long-term way of living that feeds your body and mind. Reaching your target weight is just the beginning of the road. Rather, it is the start of a new chapter in which you continue to make wise decisions, build wholesome routines, and prioritize your long-term health.

Living the South Beach lifestyle is about more than just following a diet plan—it's about cultivating a mindset that prioritizes your health. It's about understanding how food affects your body, fueling it with the right nutrients, and treating your body with the respect it deserves. As you transition from one phase to the next, remember that each step is a part of your lifelong health journey.

There will be challenges along the way. You may face social events, cravings, and obstacles that tempt you to veer off track. But the key is to stay focused on your goals and understand that every healthy choice you make is a step toward a better, healthier version of yourself.

Staying Motivated

Motivation can come and go, but the key to staying on track is to develop habits that support your health goals even when motivation dips. Here are some strategies to help you stay motivated and committed to the South Beach Diet:

- *Set Realistic Goals:* Start with small, achievable goals. These could be as simple as cooking one new South Beach-approved recipe each week or tracking your water intake daily. Celebrate your progress, even the small wins, and use them as fuel to keep going.

- *Track Your Progress:* Use a journal or an app to track your meals, workouts, and how you're feeling. Visualizing your progress can keep you inspired. These observable advantages—whether they be better digestion, increased energy, or weight loss—will serve as a reminder of why you began.

- *Focus on Non-Scale Victories:* While weight loss is often the goal, don't forget about the other positive changes happening in your body. Your energy levels, better sleep, clearer skin, and improved mood are all signs that the South Beach Diet is working for you. These victories can be just as motivating as the number on the scale.

- *Create a Routine:* Consistency is key to maintaining a healthy lifestyle. Make a timetable that suits your personal lifestyle.. Whether it's meal prepping on Sundays or setting aside time for a daily walk, having a routine can make healthy habits feel effortless.

- *Find Accountability:* Whether it's a friend, family member, or an online community, find someone or a group that can hold you accountable. Sharing your goals with others and supporting each other can provide extra motivation and encouragement.

- *Remember Why You Started:* On tough days, remind yourself of why you started this journey in the first place. Whether it's to feel better, improve your health, or achieve a specific weight goal, keeping your reasons in mind can help you push through the challenges.

The South Beach Diet is not a quick fix, but a lifestyle change that will benefit you for years to come. Motivation will ebb and flow, but as long as you stick to your routine, the results will follow.

Resources and Support

As you continue with the South Beach Diet, having the right resources and support can make a huge difference in your success. From meal planning to staying motivated, having the tools you need will help you stay on track.

- *Books and Cookbooks:* Keep a few South Beach Diet cookbooks on hand to inspire you in the kitchen. These books provide a variety of recipes that align with each phase of the diet, making it easier to find meals that fit your lifestyle and taste preferences. Cooking healthy meals doesn't have to be boring or time-consuming, and having a range of recipes at your fingertips can make sticking to the diet enjoyable.

- *Online Communities:* Joining online groups or forums where others are following the South Beach Diet can be incredibly helpful. You can find recipes, share experiences, and get advice on handling challenges. Whether it's on Facebook, Reddit, or other social platforms, connecting with people who share your goals can make the journey feel less isolating.

- *Apps and Tracking Tools:* There are several apps available that can help you track your meals, workouts, and progress. These tools allow you to stay organized and stay mindful of your food choices. Many apps also have built-in support for tracking calories, macronutrients, and other health metrics, which can help you stay aligned with the diet's guidelines.

- *Health Coaches and Nutritionists:* If you need personalized support or guidance, consider working with a health coach or nutritionist who can help you navigate the South Beach Diet. They can offer advice tailored to your specific needs and help you overcome any hurdles you might face.

- *Recipes and Meal Plans*: To make meal planning easier, use resources like meal planning websites or apps that offer weekly South Beach-friendly menus. Planning ahead can help you stay on track and prevent impulse decisions when you're hungry. A well-stocked pantry and a clear meal plan for the week can make all the difference in sticking to your goals.

- *Fitness Support:* Incorporating regular physical activity into your routine will accelerate your results and help you maintain long-term success. There are many fitness apps, YouTube channels, and online programs that cater to all levels of fitness. Whether you prefer yoga, strength training, or cardio, having a workout plan that complements your diet can help you stay motivated and achieve better results.

- *Support Groups and Forums:* Whether it's in person or online, having a support system can make a big difference. Join a local group, or seek out virtual support from people who are going through the same journey. Sharing experiences, tips, and motivation can be helpful, especially when things feel tough.

- *Regular Check-ins with Your Healthcare Provider:* It's always a good idea to check in with your healthcare provider periodically. They can help monitor your progress and ensure that you're following a plan that supports your overall health. If you have any underlying health conditions, they can guide you on how to adapt the diet for your specific needs.

Final Thoughts

The South Beach Diet offers you a simple and sustainable path to better health. It's not a quick fix but a long-term strategy that teaches you to eat smarter, feel better, and live a healthier life. Your journey is about finding balance—between the food you eat, your level of physical activity, and your mental well-being.

As you move forward, remember that there will be highs and lows. There will be days when everything feels easy and days when it's harder to stay on track. But consistency is what will get you to your goal. Stay committed, stay focused, and keep in mind that every positive change you make is a step in the right direction.

Whether you're just starting or already in maintenance mode, the South Beach Diet can help you build a foundation for a healthier, happier life. Don't be afraid to ask for support, celebrate your successes, and continue learning. With the right mindset, resources, and habits, you can make this diet work for you, not just for a few months, but for a lifetime.

A Thank You Note from Kristy Nolan

Thank you so much for choosing The South Beach Diet of 2025: The Ultimate Guide to Effortless Weight Loss Through Simple and Healthy Cooking. I'm truly grateful that you've taken this step toward better health and wellness with me. It's my hope that the tips, recipes, and strategies in this book will help you on your journey to lasting weight loss, increased energy, and a healthier lifestyle.

If you found this book helpful, I'd love for you to leave an honest review. Your feedback is important to me and helps others make an informed decision. You can have a significant impact with only a few words!

Also, be sure to check out my other books for more recipes, tips, and lifestyle guidance on staying healthy, feeling great, and maintaining your weight loss goals.

Please feel free to get in touch with me if you need any sort of help or if you have any questions! I'd be glad to assist. I can be reached at *[kristynolanbooks@gmail.com]* at any time.

Thank you again for your support, and I wish you all the best on your health journey. Keep going strong – you're doing amazing!

With gratitude,
Kristy Nolan

🎁 CLAIM YOUR EXCLUSIVE BONUSES!

Thank you for taking this important step toward better health! To access your valuable bonus package, including the Substitution Guide and Phase-by-Phase Food Lists:

- Scan the QR code on the next page using your smartphone camera
- Enter the unique code found on your book's receipt
- Download your digital bonus package instantly

Your commitment to health deserves to be rewarded. Enjoy these powerful tools to maximize your South Beach Diet success!

-Kristy Nolan

The South Beach Diet Of 2025 | 169

WEIGHT LOSS TRACKER & 30-DAYS WELLNESS TRACKER

Thank you for being a part of this journey. I congratulate you and I also appreciate you for taking a bold step by getting a copy of the South Beach Diet Book for 2025.

As a little token to show my appreciation for your purchase, here's your bonus and I hope you love it and use it to track your weight loss journey

You can do well to drop positive feedback and tell me what you think of the book in the Amazon book review section.

Thanks, my friend!

The South Beach Diet
Measurement Tracker

BEFORE	AFTER
Weight _____	Weight _____
Date _____	Date _____

BEFORE		AFTER
RIGHT ARM _____		_____ RIGHT ARM
LEFT ARM _____		_____ LEFT ARM
CGEST _____		_____ CGEST
WAIST _____		_____ WAIST
HIPS _____		_____ HIPS
RIGHT THIGH _____		_____ RIGHT THIGH
LEFT THIGH _____		_____ LEFT THIGH
RIGHT CALF _____		_____ RIGHT CALF
LEFT CALF _____		_____ LEFT CALF

NOTES

*
*

The South Beach Diet
Measurement Tracker

BEFORE | **AFTER**

Weight _____ Weight _____
Date _____ Date _____

RIGHT ARM _____ RIGHT ARM _____

LEFT ARM _____ LEFT ARM _____

CGEST _____ CGEST _____

WAIST _____ WAIST _____

HIPS _____ HIPS _____

RIGHT THIGH _____ RIGHT THIGH _____

LEFT THIGH _____ LEFT THIGH _____

RIGHT CALF _____ RIGHT CALF _____

LEFT CALF _____ LEFT CALF _____

NOTES

*
*

The South Beach Diet
Measurement Tracker

BEFORE   **AFTER**

BEFORE	AFTER
Weight _____	Weight _____
Date _____	Date _____
RIGHT ARM _____	RIGHT ARM _____
LEFT ARM _____	LEFT ARM _____
CGEST _____	CGEST _____
WAIST _____	WAIST _____
HIPS _____	HIPS _____
RIGHT THIGH _____	RIGHT THIGH _____
LEFT THIGH _____	LEFT THIGH _____
RIGHT CALF _____	RIGHT CALF _____
LEFT CALF _____	LEFT CALF _____

NOTES
*
*

The South Beach Diet Of 2025

The South Beach Diet
Measurement Tracker

BEFORE   **AFTER**

BEFORE	AFTER
Weight _____	Weight _____
Date _____	Date _____
RIGHT ARM _____	RIGHT ARM _____
LEFT ARM _____	LEFT ARM _____
CGEST _____	CGEST _____
WAIST _____	WAIST _____
HIPS _____	HIPS _____
RIGHT THIGH _____	RIGHT THIGH _____
LEFT THIGH _____	LEFT THIGH _____
RIGHT CALF _____	RIGHT CALF _____
LEFT CALF _____	LEFT CALF _____

NOTES

*
*

The South Beach Diet
Measurement Tracker

BEFORE   **AFTER**

Weight _____   Weight _____

Date _____   Date _____

RIGHT ARM _____   _____ **RIGHT ARM**

LEFT ARM _____   _____ **LEFT ARM**

CGEST _____   _____ **CGEST**

WAIST _____   _____ **WAIST**

HIPS _____   _____ **HIPS**

RIGHT THIGH _____   _____ **RIGHT THIGH**

LEFT THIGH _____   _____ **LEFT THIGH**

RIGHT CALF _____   _____ **RIGHT CALF**

LEFT CALF _____   _____ **LEFT CALF**

NOTES

*
*

The South Beach Diet
Measurement Tracker

BEFORE   **AFTER**

BEFORE	AFTER
Weight _____	Weight _____
Date _____	Date _____
RIGHT ARM _____	RIGHT ARM _____
LEFT ARM _____	LEFT ARM _____
CGEST _____	CGEST _____
WAIST _____	WAIST _____
HIPS _____	HIPS _____
RIGHT THIGH _____	RIGHT THIGH _____
LEFT THIGH _____	LEFT THIGH _____
RIGHT CALF _____	RIGHT CALF _____
LEFT CALF _____	LEFT CALF _____

NOTES

*
*

30 Day Wellness Tracker

MONTH: _____

SLEEP

DAY 1	DAY 2	DAY 3	DAY 4	DAY 5	DAY 6	DAY 7	DAY 8	DAY 9	DAY 10
DAY 11	DAY 12	DAY 13	DAY 14	DAY 15	DAY 16	DAY 17	DAY 18	DAY 19	DAY 20
DAY 21	DAY 22	DAY 23	DAY 24	DAY 25	DAY 26	DAY 27	DAY 28	DAY 29	DAY 30

SELF CARE ROUTINE

DAY 1	DAY 2	DAY 3	DAY 4	DAY 5	DAY 6	DAY 7	DAY 8	DAY 9	DAY 10
DAY 11	DAY 12	DAY 13	DAY 14	DAY 15	DAY 16	DAY 17	DAY 18	DAY 19	DAY 20
DAY 21	DAY 22	DAY 23	DAY 24	DAY 25	DAY 26	DAY 27	DAY 28	DAY 29	DAY 30

EXERCISE

DAY 1	DAY 2	DAY 3	DAY 4	DAY 5	DAY 6	DAY 7	DAY 8	DAY 9	DAY 10
DAY 11	DAY 12	DAY 13	DAY 14	DAY 15	DAY 16	DAY 17	DAY 18	DAY 19	DAY 20
DAY 21	DAY 22	DAY 23	DAY 24	DAY 25	DAY 26	DAY 27	DAY 28	DAY 29	DAY 30

MEAL PLAN

DAY 1	DAY 2	DAY 3	DAY 4	DAY 5	DAY 6	DAY 7	DAY 8	DAY 9	DAY 10
DAY 11	DAY 12	DAY 13	DAY 14	DAY 15	DAY 16	DAY 17	DAY 18	DAY 19	DAY 20
DAY 21	DAY 22	DAY 23	DAY 24	DAY 25	DAY 26	DAY 27	DAY 28	DAY 29	DAY 30

30 Day Wellness Tracker

MONTH: _____

SLEEP

DAY 1	DAY 2	DAY 3	DAY 4	DAY 5	DAY 6	DAY 7	DAY 8	DAY 9	DAY 10
DAY 11	DAY 12	DAY 13	DAY 14	DAY 15	DAY 16	DAY 17	DAY 18	DAY 19	DAY 20
DAY 21	DAY 22	DAY 23	DAY 24	DAY 25	DAY 26	DAY 27	DAY 28	DAY 29	DAY 30

SELF CARE ROUTINE

DAY 1	DAY 2	DAY 3	DAY 4	DAY 5	DAY 6	DAY 7	DAY 8	DAY 9	DAY 10
DAY 11	DAY 12	DAY 13	DAY 14	DAY 15	DAY 16	DAY 17	DAY 18	DAY 19	DAY 20
DAY 21	DAY 22	DAY 23	DAY 24	DAY 25	DAY 26	DAY 27	DAY 28	DAY 29	DAY 30

EXERCISE

DAY 1	DAY 2	DAY 3	DAY 4	DAY 5	DAY 6	DAY 7	DAY 8	DAY 9	DAY 10
DAY 11	DAY 12	DAY 13	DAY 14	DAY 15	DAY 16	DAY 17	DAY 18	DAY 19	DAY 20
DAY 21	DAY 22	DAY 23	DAY 24	DAY 25	DAY 26	DAY 27	DAY 28	DAY 29	DAY 30

MEAL PLAN

DAY 1	DAY 2	DAY 3	DAY 4	DAY 5	DAY 6	DAY 7	DAY 8	DAY 9	DAY 10
DAY 11	DAY 12	DAY 13	DAY 14	DAY 15	DAY 16	DAY 17	DAY 18	DAY 19	DAY 20
DAY 21	DAY 22	DAY 23	DAY 24	DAY 25	DAY 26	DAY 27	DAY 28	DAY 29	DAY 30

30 Day Wellness Tracker

MONTH: _____

SLEEP

DAY 1	DAY 2	DAY 3	DAY 4	DAY 5	DAY 6	DAY 7	DAY 8	DAY 9	DAY 10
DAY 11	DAY 12	DAY 13	DAY 14	DAY 15	DAY 16	DAY 17	DAY 18	DAY 19	DAY 20
DAY 21	DAY 22	DAY 23	DAY 24	DAY 25	DAY 26	DAY 27	DAY 28	DAY 29	DAY 30

SELF CARE ROUTINE

DAY 1	DAY 2	DAY 3	DAY 4	DAY 5	DAY 6	DAY 7	DAY 8	DAY 9	DAY 10
DAY 11	DAY 12	DAY 13	DAY 14	DAY 15	DAY 16	DAY 17	DAY 18	DAY 19	DAY 20
DAY 21	DAY 22	DAY 23	DAY 24	DAY 25	DAY 26	DAY 27	DAY 28	DAY 29	DAY 30

EXERCISE

DAY 1	DAY 2	DAY 3	DAY 4	DAY 5	DAY 6	DAY 7	DAY 8	DAY 9	DAY 10
DAY 11	DAY 12	DAY 13	DAY 14	DAY 15	DAY 16	DAY 17	DAY 18	DAY 19	DAY 20
DAY 21	DAY 22	DAY 23	DAY 24	DAY 25	DAY 26	DAY 27	DAY 28	DAY 29	DAY 30

MEAL PLAN

DAY 1	DAY 2	DAY 3	DAY 4	DAY 5	DAY 6	DAY 7	DAY 8	DAY 9	DAY 10
DAY 11	DAY 12	DAY 13	DAY 14	DAY 15	DAY 16	DAY 17	DAY 18	DAY 19	DAY 20
DAY 21	DAY 22	DAY 23	DAY 24	DAY 25	DAY 26	DAY 27	DAY 28	DAY 29	DAY 30

30 Day Wellness Tracker

MONTH: _____

SLEEP

DAY 1	DAY 2	DAY 3	DAY 4	DAY 5	DAY 6	DAY 7	DAY 8	DAY 9	DAY 10
DAY 11	DAY 12	DAY 13	DAY 14	DAY 15	DAY 16	DAY 17	DAY 18	DAY 19	DAY 20
DAY 21	DAY 22	DAY 23	DAY 24	DAY 25	DAY 26	DAY 27	DAY 28	DAY 29	DAY 30

SELF CARE ROUTINE

DAY 1	DAY 2	DAY 3	DAY 4	DAY 5	DAY 6	DAY 7	DAY 8	DAY 9	DAY 10
DAY 11	DAY 12	DAY 13	DAY 14	DAY 15	DAY 16	DAY 17	DAY 18	DAY 19	DAY 20
DAY 21	DAY 22	DAY 23	DAY 24	DAY 25	DAY 26	DAY 27	DAY 28	DAY 29	DAY 30

EXERCISE

DAY 1	DAY 2	DAY 3	DAY 4	DAY 5	DAY 6	DAY 7	DAY 8	DAY 9	DAY 10
DAY 11	DAY 12	DAY 13	DAY 14	DAY 15	DAY 16	DAY 17	DAY 18	DAY 19	DAY 20
DAY 21	DAY 22	DAY 23	DAY 24	DAY 25	DAY 26	DAY 27	DAY 28	DAY 29	DAY 30

MEAL PLAN

DAY 1	DAY 2	DAY 3	DAY 4	DAY 5	DAY 6	DAY 7	DAY 8	DAY 9	DAY 10
DAY 11	DAY 12	DAY 13	DAY 14	DAY 15	DAY 16	DAY 17	DAY 18	DAY 19	DAY 20
DAY 21	DAY 22	DAY 23	DAY 24	DAY 25	DAY 26	DAY 27	DAY 28	DAY 29	DAY 30

30 Day Wellness Tracker

MONTH: _____

SLEEP

DAY 1	DAY 2	DAY 3	DAY 4	DAY 5	DAY 6	DAY 7	DAY 8	DAY 9	DAY 10
DAY 11	DAY 12	DAY 13	DAY 14	DAY 15	DAY 16	DAY 17	DAY 18	DAY 19	DAY 20
DAY 21	DAY 22	DAY 23	DAY 24	DAY 25	DAY 26	DAY 27	DAY 28	DAY 29	DAY 30

SELF CARE ROUTINE

DAY 1	DAY 2	DAY 3	DAY 4	DAY 5	DAY 6	DAY 7	DAY 8	DAY 9	DAY 10
DAY 11	DAY 12	DAY 13	DAY 14	DAY 15	DAY 16	DAY 17	DAY 18	DAY 19	DAY 20
DAY 21	DAY 22	DAY 23	DAY 24	DAY 25	DAY 26	DAY 27	DAY 28	DAY 29	DAY 30

EXERCISE

DAY 1	DAY 2	DAY 3	DAY 4	DAY 5	DAY 6	DAY 7	DAY 8	DAY 9	DAY 10
DAY 11	DAY 12	DAY 13	DAY 14	DAY 15	DAY 16	DAY 17	DAY 18	DAY 19	DAY 20
DAY 21	DAY 22	DAY 23	DAY 24	DAY 25	DAY 26	DAY 27	DAY 28	DAY 29	DAY 30

MEAL PLAN

DAY 1	DAY 2	DAY 3	DAY 4	DAY 5	DAY 6	DAY 7	DAY 8	DAY 9	DAY 10
DAY 11	DAY 12	DAY 13	DAY 14	DAY 15	DAY 16	DAY 17	DAY 18	DAY 19	DAY 20
DAY 21	DAY 22	DAY 23	DAY 24	DAY 25	DAY 26	DAY 27	DAY 28	DAY 29	DAY 30

Check out my other books on Amazon by scanning the QR Code below and also check out other books of mine on the Keto diet and South Beach Diet.

THE SOUTH BEACH DIET OF 2024

HEALTHY WEIGHTLOSS FAST

THE ULTIMATE GUIDE TO EFFORTLESS AND HEALTHY WEIGHT LOSS FOR IMPROVED HEALTH

KRISTY NOLAN

KETO DIET COOKBOOK for BEGINNERS 2024

7-WEEKS MEAL PLANNER

28 DAYS MEAL PLAN

Kristy Nolan

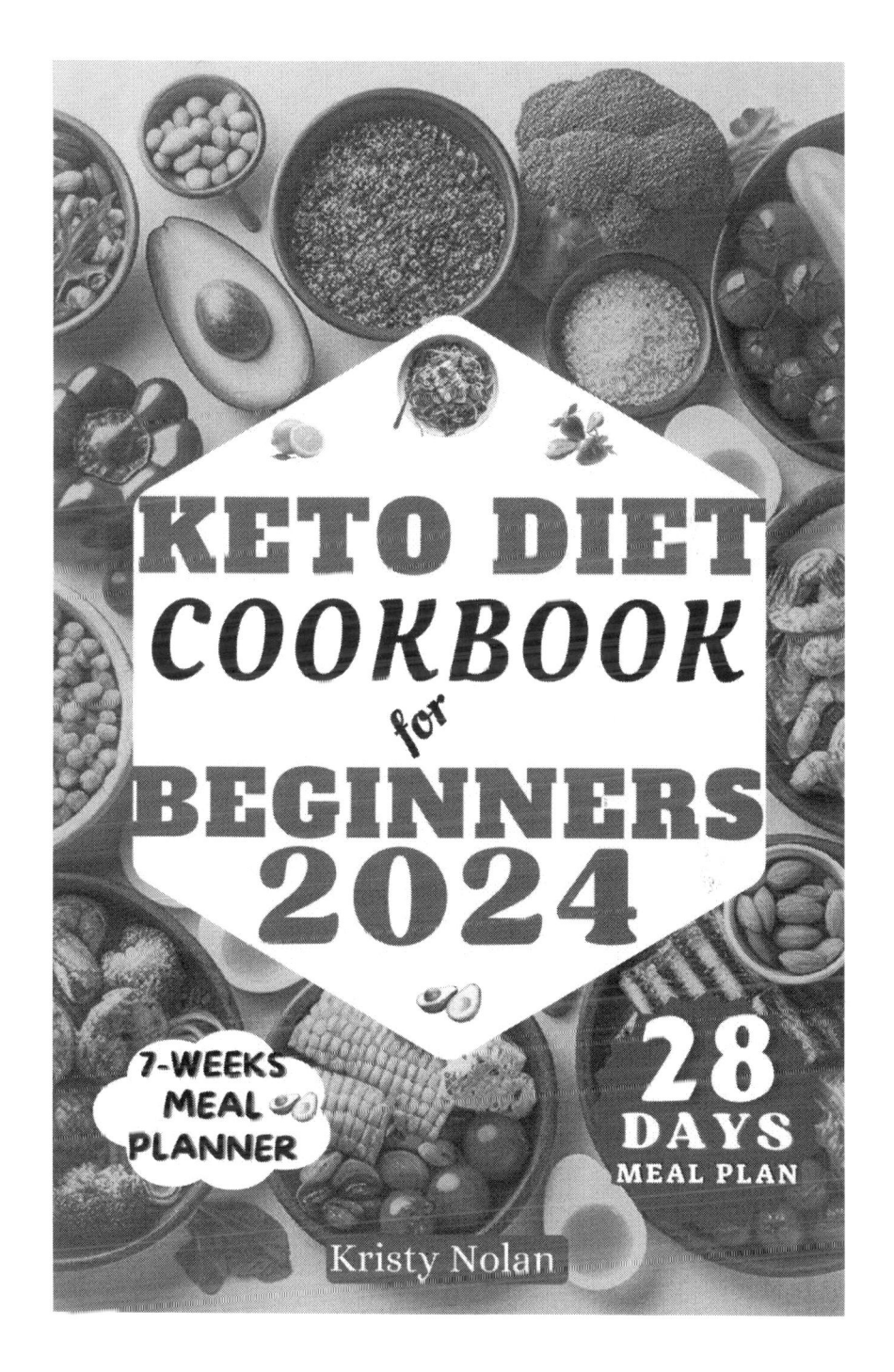

THE SOUTH BEACH DIET COOKBOOK 2024

Quick and Easy Recipes

PLUS COMPLETE GUIDE TO HELP LOSE WEIGHT FAST

KRISTY NOLAN

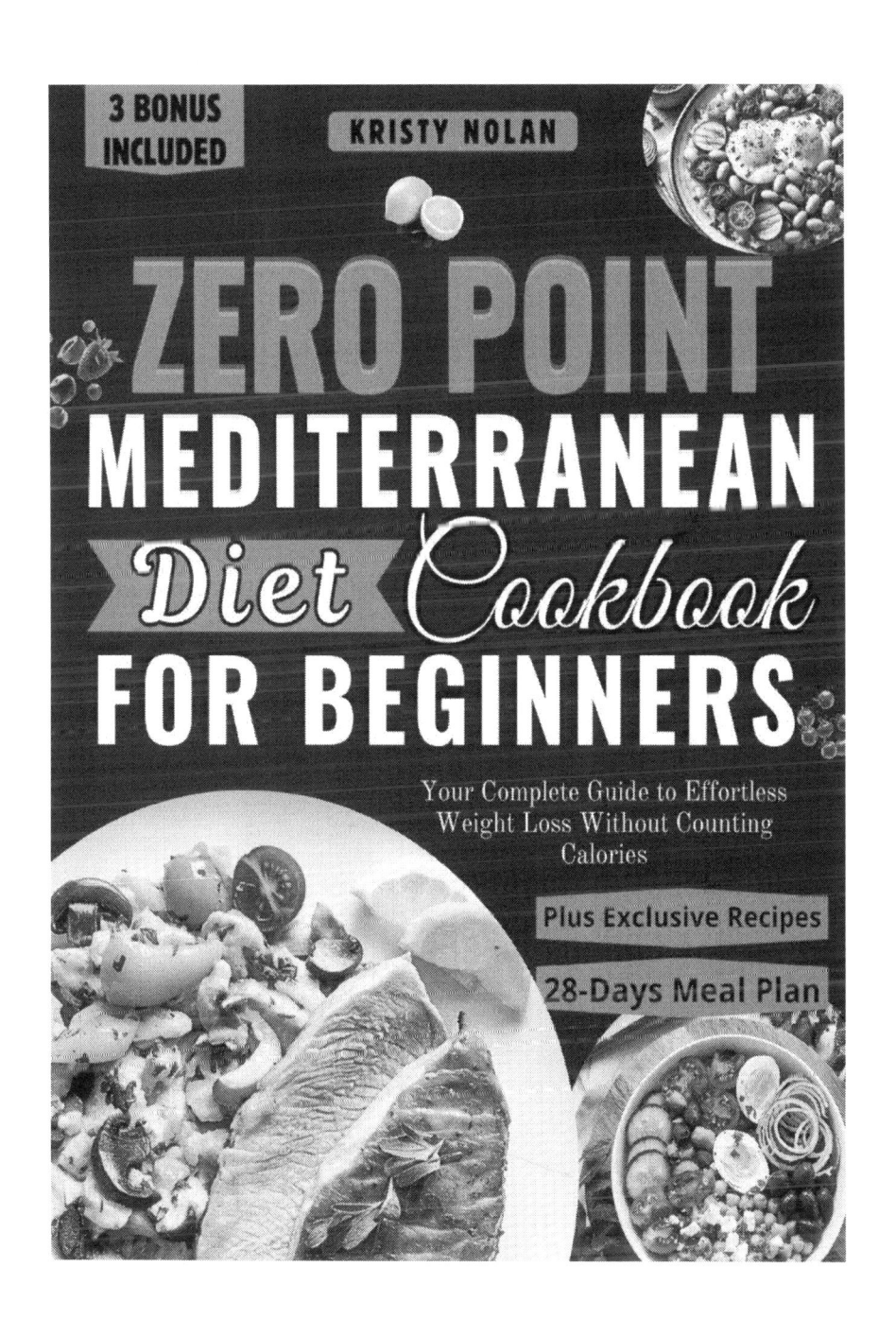

ZERO POINT MEDITERRANEAN Diet Cookbook FOR BEGINNERS

3 BONUS INCLUDED

KRISTY NOLAN

Your Complete Guide to Effortless Weight Loss Without Counting Calories

Plus Exclusive Recipes

28-Days Meal Plan

THE SOUTH BEACH DIET COOKBOOK 2023

Plus Delicious Recipes

QUICK AND EASY RECIPES IN 30 MINUTES TO LOSE WEIGHT FAST

KRISTY NOLAN

Made in the USA
Middletown, DE
08 July 2025